HEALTHY LIVING *by Design*

A new you is waiting

YOUR 6 WEEK GUIDE TO WELLNESS TRANSFORMATION

LINDA K. MCCLEAD

Health, Wellness & Lifestyle Coach

Healthy Living by Design

Your 6 Week Guide to Wellness Transformation

Copyright © 2017 by Linda K. McClead

This book contains the opinions, ideas, and beliefs of the author. It is intended to provide information and suggestions to improve the quality of life for those who are seeking to make positive lifestyle changes. If the reader requires personal health, medical, psychological, or any other personal professional services, a competent professional should be consulted. The author and publisher specifically disclaims all responsibility for any loss, liability, or risk, personal or otherwise, that is incurred as a consequence, directly or indirectly, of the use and application of any of the contents of this book.

Before beginning any fitness or weight loss program, always check with your physician to make sure that the changes are appropriate and safe for you. Due to possible interactions with medicines or health conditions, consult your physician before adding supplements, herbs, or new foods to your lifestyle.

All rights reserved. No part of this book may be reproduced in any form or by any electronic or mechanical means, including information storage and retrieval systems, without permission in writing from the author.

To contact Linda McClead:

lindalivingbydesign@gmail.com

healthylivingbydesign.liveeditaurora.com

ISBN-10: 1545195722

ISBN-13: 978-1545195727

Printed in the United States of America

TABLE OF CONTENTS

Dedications	7
My Inspiration	9
Acknowledgements	11
Foreword	13
What People are Saying About Healthy Living by Design	14
Ways to use Healthy Living by Design	16
Introduction	17
My Story	19

CHAPTER 1 - LET'S BEGIN — 21

Let's Begin! Take Charge of Your Life, Starting Today	21
Desire, Commitment, Plan, Payoff	21
Success Tips	22
10 Commandments for Ultimate Health	23
Your Health Affirmation	25
Life Satisfaction Survey	28
Goal Setting	29
Chapter 1 Recap	33

CHAPTER 2 - WEEK 1 — 35

Day 1: Kitchen Clean Up	35
Day 2: New Kitchen Basics	36
Day 3: Power in Planning and Preparation	39
Day 4: Move It!	42
Day 5: Log it!	46
Day 6: Hydrate for Health	47
Day 7: Go for Greens	49
Chapter 2 Recap	51

CHAPTER 3 - WEEK 2 — 53

Day 1: Lean Protein Power	53
Day 2: Healthy Fats are Where It's At!	54
Day 3: Complex Smart Carbs	57
Day 4: Strength and Tone Zone	59
Day 5: Gratitude Attitude	60
Day 6: Dive in for Better Digestion	61
Day 7: Weight Loss Wonders	64
Chapter 3 Recap	67

CHAPTER 4 - WEEK 3   69

Day 1: Ultimate Health Food Diary, Tips, & Logging   69
Day 2: Grains   75
Day 3: Immune Boosting with Superfoods and Antioxidants   78
Day 4: Fitness Tips for Maximum Calorie Burn   81
Day 5: Journaling Basics – Morning and Evening   84
Day 6: Home Cooking   88
Day 7: Breakfast Magic   90
Chapter 4 Recap   93

CHAPTER 5 - WEEK 4   95

Day 1: Disease Prevention   95
Day 2: Healthful Teas, Super Spices and More   100
Day 3: Feed your Soul-Nurture your Spirit   102
Day 4: Calming Exercises to Feed the Soul   106
Day 5: Anti-Aging   112
Day 6: Stress Less   114
Day 7: Be Happy   120
Chapter 5 Recap   124

CHAPTER 6 - WEEK 5   127

Day 1: Soothing Sleep   127
Day 2: Serving Sizes and Portion Control   130
Day 3: Healthy Eating When Dining Out   132
Day 4: Simple Fitness Assessments   134
Day 5: Numbers to Know   135
Day 6: Your Physical Environment   137
Day 7: Alternative Healing Modalities   140
Chapter 6 Recap   146

CHAPTER 7 - WEEK 6   149

Day 1: Detoxification   149
Day 2: Relationships   150
Day 3: Individualize Your Plan   154
Day 4: Fit for Life   155
Day 5: Time Management & Priorities   157
Day 6: Find your Joy, Purpose and Passion   159
Day 7: Life Review and Refining your Goals   163
Chapter 7 Recap   170

RESOURCES 173

Holistic Approach to Health 173
Grocery Store List 174
Healthy Snack Foods List 176
Sample 3 Day Food Plan 178
Goal Setting Suggestions 181
My Wishes for You 183

Index 185

DEDICATIONS

My Grandmother and Mother

My grandmother, Thelma Roberts was my mentor and inspiration in life. She taught me to work hard and to find a purpose and passion so that my life would be fulfilling and meaningful. By her example, I'm living my life attempting to enhance the quality of life of others. She taught me to share what I know and be of service and of value.

At age 58, she earned her Master's Degree.

And now, at age 58, I'm realizing my dream of publishing my book.

I hope you are proud, Gran. I love you. I miss you every day.

My Mother, Betty Nulter, taught me the importance of friendship, laughter, and that happiness is found in the simple everyday things in life.

My Children

To my three wonderful children - Megan, Molly and Matthew

    It is truly an honor to be your Mother.

    The three of you are my greatest gifts and my greatest joy!

My Grandchildren

Gage, Jake, Macie, and Owen

    I adore you!

    I plan to feed you better than I did your parents!

    Maybe I will throw some broccoli in your cupcakes!

    But don't worry, you'll love it!

YOU!

Last, but not least, this book is dedicated to you, the reader!

    I pray that this book will be the catalyst and inspiration that you need to make yourself a priority!

    I hope it will put you on a more positive path.

    If you are ready to make lifestyle changes, I'm here to help.

    If your desire is to have a more rewarding, happy, healthy life, this book is for you!

MY INSPIRATION

The inspiration for this book was my quest for knowledge and information to better the lives of my family members as well as myself. Our family genetics involve a lot of health issues and disease. Knowledge is truly power. Doing research and learning how to optimize my health and reduce disease risks gave me the control to do something about some of those concerns. I know it will help you and your family too.

Our lifestyle choices greatly influence our health.

The older we get, the more we realize this. It is never too late to take care of yourself and create new healthier habits to live better, longer, and happier.

This isn't a diet. It is a new way of life.

One that will focus on yourself.
You will learn to make yourself a priority and practice extreme self-care.

How the Book came to Life

The book came about gradually over many years. I began to teach graduate classes for West Virginia University in 2007. The first class was a group fitness class with some emphasis on diet and lifestyle. As time went on, I began to add more and more wellness related topics to the course until it took a much more holistic approach to healthy living.

Finally, I realized that instead of giving so many handouts, I should compile the content into a book to use for the class. The first draft of the book was printed locally in 2010.

In 2012, I began working at Camden Clark Health and Wellness Center as a fitness coordinator, instructor and health coach. It is there that I began teaching the Wellness Transformation Program, Weight Loss Programs and Group Personal Training Programs for the community. *Healthy Living by Design* is the workbook and guide that I use to teach the small group Wellness Transformation Classes.

In 2017 I am realizing my goal to re-organize and update the book so that it can be used as a self-help and informational book by anyone to use on their own to make healthy changes. I also will continue to use the book for my small group programs.

ACKNOWLEDGEMENTS

Institute for Integrative Nutrition

One of the smartest decisions I've made was enrolling in the comprehensive health coaching program at the Institute for Integrative Nutrition. Because of this program, my personal health, career, and positive impact on my friends and family have been enhanced. The knowledge and insight that I gained through this program was invaluable. I was given the information and confidence to make health and wellness my life's work. My main goal is to assist people in improving the quality of their lives.

As I write this book, I am receiving guidance from an additional course from the Institute for Integrative Nutrition. It is called, "Launch Your Dream Book". The path and tools I'm learning from this course have helped me to make publishing my book possible. Special thanks to my accountability partner, Debbie Stoltz for your encouragement, insight and caring. Nothing happens by accident. Debbie and I were meant to cross paths. Our stories are so similar, it is unbelievable. Thank you, Debbie, for the love and light you've brought into my world.

You may be interested in the Health Coach Training Program from IIN. Some people enroll in the program for the sole purpose of reaching optimal health, wellness and balance for themselves and their families. After completing the program, you may decide to become a health coach. Besides the health coach training program, IIN offers courses in business, marketing, and book publishing. If you are interested in pursuing IIN and seeing if it is right for you, contact me. I'd be happy to help. You can contact me at lindalivingbydesign@gmail.com or healthylivingbydesign.liveeditaurora.com

Thank you to my family and friends for your love, encouragement and support:

Megan, Molly, Matthew

Lanita, Patty, Ray, Roc, Katrina, Glenna, Peggy

Graduate Class Students from West Virginia University/RESA V

David Hawkins, Master Herbalist and Owner of Mother Earth Foods

Clients and Participants in my Fitness, Wellness and Weight Loss Programs

West Virginia University Medicine-Camden Clark Health and Wellness Center Staff

FOREWARD

Healthy Living by Design
will provide you with information, knowledge, and tools
to make improvements in all areas of your life:

Body, Mind, Spirit, Environment, and Relationship

You will learn to make more deliberate, informed choices.

Focusing on your well-being will lead you to a happier and healthier life.

"Linda's book will help you to realize that the most important relationship you have is the one you have with yourself. With her motivation and inspiration, you will begin to make yourself a priority and practice extreme self-care. Everyone around you will benefit from a less stressed and healthier you.

Linda will guide you to set goals and make choices to design a wonderful future for yourself and your loved ones. This Wellness Transformation Program will assist you in implementing healthy lifestyle changes to make your life the best that it can be! Linda makes change fun and doable. No more dieting or deprivation.

I've known Linda for several decades. I've been both a co-worker and a student in her courses. I've witnessed literally hundreds of people make improvements in their lives through Linda's classes and programs. She is the real deal. Let her be your guide to re-write a happier, healthier ending to your life story.

I am a fitness instructor, but Linda taught me that being fit is much more than just exercising. It encompasses your total body, mind, and spirit. It was wonderful to have an instructor that loves what they are teaching, is passionate about helping people, and conveys such an important message for life. She teaches you to be good to yourself so that you can be more fully present for others. Her knowledge and expertise I can count on and believe in to help guide me and my family on our journey to healthy living."

-Lanita Wentzel

Read on to see what other recent clients had to say about Linda's programs:

WHAT PEOPLE ARE SAYING ABOUT
HEALTHY LIVING BY DESIGN...

"I am a wife and a mother of 5 children. I have a very hectic life keeping up with my family and everyday life. Linda was able to teach me that it is ok to take time out for myself and that I need to do things that benefit me. I didn't realize that I was always looking to make everyone else happy and full of life but that I put myself on the back burner. Putting things down on paper made things much clearer for me. I do go back and look at the goals I created with Linda's help, and it reminds me of what I need in my life. My views on life have changed, thanks to Linda."

-Maria

"What a blessing to have been able to participate in this program of yours. You have inspired and motivated me to think healthy every day, truly, and make wise choices. Thank you for providing an abundance of information and suggested methods to utilize in my continued journey toward my optimal health and well-being."

- Glenna

"As an educator, I took Linda's graduate class for credit. I learned valuable information to make necessary changes in my life. A couple years later as a "middle aged woman re-evaluating my life", I knew I needed her motivational enthusiasm to get me back on track. I was privileged to be a part of her class with her as my life coach. Not only does she inspire one to progress in their own life, but she manages to motivate one to share the wonderful tools she provides and see others reap the benefits of living a life by design. I can hear her positive and encouraging words cheer me on as I keep moving forward on the path I've chosen to pursue with the tools and inspiration she has provided."

-Jo Ellen

"Having Linda as a health coach was a fabulous experience. She is real! She had her own personal history with the subjects that we discussed in class. This ranged from unhealthy eating habits in the past to lack of personal time. Working with Linda was beneficial in every way possible. I walked away from this class healthier, happier and with a life more in balance."

-Angela

"This program is just what I needed to get started on the right path. I am ever grateful to Linda for inspiring me to take charge of my life!"

-Mindy

"By sharing her extensive knowledge, Linda has equipped me for this new journey I am on. I'm inspired to make a commitment to myself to eat healthier and shed some unwanted pounds. Linda's individual style of coaching is rare."

-Barbara

"Linda instills in you a desire to be the best you can be. She makes learning new and healthy choices for your life fun and doable. She gives you the knowledge and tools to design a healthier, happier you. Linda provides support and encouragement."

-Angie

"I felt it was a great and very educational class. Snacks were delicious…food/activity diary are great…motivating…Linda's grasp of subject material and enthusiastic attitude and ability to communicate are big plusses."

-Chuck

WAYS TO USE HEALTHY LIVING BY DESIGN

How to use this book on your own:

In Chapter One you will receive the needed background knowledge, motivation and preparation that you will need to move forward on your quest for making new lifestyle changes.

Then, beginning with Chapter Two, each chapter will have 7 sections, one for each day of the week. Simply read one section daily and incorporate the new lifestyle changes and additions to your life. Over a 6 -week period, you will develop knowledge, tips and tools to make many permanent healthy changes.

Wellness Facility Trainer, Life Coach, Health Coach or Nutritionist:

Individuals working in fitness, weight loss or nutrition fields can use the book as a guide to facilitate your own 6- week Wellness Transformation Program.

Colleges and Universities:

Healthy Living by Design could also be used at colleges to offer graduate classes for teachers for certification renewal or as an elective course in any health -related field. I currently offer a graduate class for West Virginia University.

Churches:

Churches often have a "healthy lifestyle" class or club. This book will provide the format for a program for your Sunday School Class or on-going program.

Fitness Certification Organizations:

Another way the book could be used is for fitness certification organizations to use it as the guide for wellness coach certification course offerings.

Corporations, Schools, Churches, Hospitals, or Other Facilities:

Hire Linda to speak at your next event or to hold a workshops or program for your organization.

Linda has been helping clients achieve better heath, wellness and quality of life for many years. She speaks to groups and organizations on a variety of wellness topics. Sample topics include: Holistic Healthy Habits, Eating for Energy, How to Stress Less, Weight Loss Tips and Tricks, Finding your Purpose and Passion, Sleep, Rest, & Relaxation, Wellness Transformation Tips and Lifestyle Changes for Health.

INTRODUCTION

Healthy Living by Design will provide the roadmap that you need to create new healthy habits for life. The tips, tools and information you will receive will help you to focus on yourself and learn how to practice great self-care. Living a happy, healthy life includes paying attention to all aspects of life and choosing to make deliberate goals and decisions that are beneficial to your mind, body, and spirit.

I want to show you how to make yourself a priority and design a life that is full of health, joy, peace, and contentment. My mission with this book is to assist you in making more conscious and healthy choices to enhance the quality of your life.

What you put in your body is crucial for disease prevention and longevity. Eating healthfully will enable your immune system to work efficiently and fight off disease. You will have more energy and vitality. You will be amazed with how the quality of the food you eat affects how you feel both physically and emotionally.

In addition to making changes in the food that you eat, I'll teach you how to make changes in all areas of your life. My Wellness Transformation Plan will enable you to make slow and steady progress as you incorporate many permanent lifestyle changes into your routine. I am not advocating a diet. This is simply a new path you will be undertaking to slowly create new habits that you will maintain forever. You will feel so good, that you will always want to maintain your new healthy lifestyle.

Chapter one will provide background information and get you motivated and prepared to begin. Starting with chapter 2, every day for 6 weeks you will read one daily segment and incorporate the knowledge and tips into your daily life. The end of the book has a *Resource* section with a healthy grocery list, healthy snack food list, a sample 3-day meal plan, goal setting suggestions, and my wishes for you.

I encourage you to make the commitment to make healthy changes in your life. A wonderful bonus will be that as you make positive and healthful choices, you will impact the lives of your friends and family as well. Good luck! I wish you well on the journey ahead.

Make yourself a priority. Focus on yourself and how to take very good care of your health from the inside out. You will reap great benefits as you begin to make deliberate and conscious choices that will result in you feeling the best you've ever felt.

> *"Life isn't about finding yourself.*
> *Life is about creating yourself."*
> –George Bernard Shaw

Read on to enhance your life – a Happier, Healthier You is Waiting.

MY STORY

As a young adult, I began teaching fitness classes. Throughout my life, I have been an exercise enthusiast. Honestly, it is my stress reducer. In my younger years, I was one of those lucky people who could eat about anything and not gain weight. However, in my 30's this began to catch up with me! I've done what most of us do. I've gained about 10 pounds a decade since my 30's. A few years ago, I was appalled to realize that I weighed more than I did before giving birth to twins back in 1982! Yikes!

Although the fitness piece of wellness is something I always did well, until a few years ago, I certainly did not have a handle on the nutrition aspect! I am a binge eater and I seek food for comfort as many of us do. My favorite traditions and family memories are centered around food. My 3 children and I used to sit over a half gallon of ice cream with 4 spoons and have ourselves a little party. Our favorite breakfast was brownies and Diet Pepsi. Did I know better? Yes, but it was my reality. I'm not proud of this, but once I ate a pan of fudge. The whole thing at one time. Yep, that's me. I won't mention the dozen donut incident. I was the kid who ran to the dessert table first at a church social! You get the picture.

We all must have a trigger…a reason for making change. Mine is health issues in my family and genetic history. Making lifestyle changes for health is very personal to me, as I'm sure it is for you. Heart disease, diabetes and cancer are prevalent in my family. Many of my immediate family have died in their 40's and 50's. My father died at 42 from lung cancer and my mother lost her 8-year battle with cancer in April of 2017. My only sibling died in recent years at age 59 from complications of diabetes. Many other family members are very unhealthy. I began to understand that for disease prevention, I needed to not only exercise, but change my eating and lifestyle habits.

My grandson Jake was diagnosed with autism at a young age. I began to research food, lifestyle and environmental changes that we should make for his benefit. I've spent a lot of time and energy researching cancer prevention and management too. I have learned so much about optimizing our immune system. It hit home with me that if food additives, colorings, preservatives, GMO's, pesticides, toxins, chemicals and antibiotics in our water, food and environment were not good for autism or cancer patients, they are not good for anyone.

As a fitness instructor, health coach and instructor of wellness courses for WVU and my local community, my objective is to teach and model self-care principles and moderation in all things. A holistic approach is key. Quality nutrition, stress management, sleep, relationships, environment, home-cooking, experiencing more energy, appreciating nature, simplifying, anti-aging principles and extreme self-care are examples of what I assist people with.

I have truly found my calling at age 58! I recently retired from my full-time job to focus solely in the field of health and wellness. I love my work as a health coach. I love the satisfaction that I get from teaching folks like you how to practice self-care and how to incorporate many lifestyle changes into your routine so that you can really feel your very best. Let me show you how to make more deliberate, conscious, healthy choices.

CHAPTER 1 - LET'S BEGIN

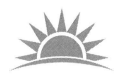

TAKE CHARGE OF YOUR LIFE, STARTING TODAY

"Life is the Sum of all your Choices"

-Albert Camus

Read the 4 steps below to begin your Wellness Transformation Journey:

Desire, Commitment, Plan, Payoff

1. Step one is simply having the desire to make healthy changes. Do you want to feel better, look better, reach your ideal weight and have more energy than you have ever had before? The fact that you had any interest in this book tells me that the answer is YES!

2. Secondly, to transform your health and wellness, you must make a commitment to make daily healthy lifestyle changes.

3. Next, you need to have a plan. I'm providing you with the plan! Starting with chapter 2, you will read one section daily and simply incorporate the new knowledge, tips and lifestyle changes into your daily life.

4. You must identify your reasons WHY you desire change! What is your payoff and ultimate goal? Identifying this will give you more motivation and determination. It will also provide focus to your transformation plan.

Some reasons why we want change are listed below. Circle the ones that you identify with.

Look Better	Feel Better	Fit into my clothes more comfortably
Feel more desirable	Improve Health	Boost Energy
Lose Weight	Have a Better Quality of Life	Tone Muscles
Feel More Confident	Other_____	

Success Tips

Success Tip 1: Make the commitment to yourself to whole heartedly begin this wellness transformation journey. **Tell your friends and family about it.** This will make you more accountable. Make a **promise to yourself** to make your health your priority right now, today.

Success Tip 2: Surround yourself with friends and family members who will support you on your health journey. Think about encouraging a co-worker or friend to begin a health transformation with you. You could even form a healthy lifestyles group at work or at church to give each other support and encouragement.

    a. Your **accountability partner** can shop with you, do food prep with you, cook with you, or share cooking responsibilities.

    b. They can eat lunch or dinner with you. Lean on each other! **Encourage each other!**

No promise is as important as the ones you make to yourself.
You can do this!

TEN COMMANDMENTS FOR ULTIMATE HEALTH

1. **Exercise your body. Treat it well.**

    Suggested guidelines: cardio 30 min 5 days per week and strength 30 minutes per week.
    Balance work and play. Make time daily for fun, play, and laughter.
    Respect and love your body. Every decision has a consequence.

2. **Exercise your mind.**

    Read, do puzzles, play games, take a class, limit "mindless activities" (TV, internet, social media).

3. **Nurture your spirit.**

    Motivational or inspirational readings, quotes, pictures, meditation, solitude, time outdoors in fresh air and sunshine, journaling, affirmations, positive self-talk, a pleasing environment.

4. **Eat, drink, and be jolly....in moderation.**

    Follow the ultimate health food plan to be sure to get a variety of healthy foods. Strive to make more home cooked meals, limit "fast food", and avoid empty calorie, processed foods.

5. **Live in the present.**

    Enjoy the now....forgive the past and look forward to the future. Let go of guilt and regret. Create the future that you want to have…it is never too late.

6. **Set goals…make changes to be happier and healthier.**

    Make a "to do" list weekly, make a bucket list, set fitness, nutrition, personal and professional goals. Make a plan to make those goals happen. Do something every day toward achieving your dreams. Empower yourself to make your health and wellness your priority.

7. **Take care of your physical health.**

    Get a primary care physician and have appropriate tests and screenings as advised. Keep a file of your health information and numbers. Make a living will and have a friend or family member be your health advocate, get quality sleep, and manage your stress.

8. **Develop a strong support system. Nurture your relationships.**

    Make time for close friends and family. Consider adopting a pet from your local animal shelter. Make sure your career, family, friends and activities feed and inspire you, instead of draining your energy. Get connected! Join a club. Take a class. Find a hobby you enjoy. Be more social.

9. **Indulge in pampering activities for yourself each week!**

   Massage, sauna, movie or lunch with a friend, take a class, listen to music, read, draw, and paint. Do something every day that makes you feel alive and happy!

10. **Be of service to others. Give of your time, energy, knowledge, and resources.**

    Focus on others…make it a goal every day to make someone else's day. Share what you know. Make sure the people in your life know how much they are appreciated, loved, and valued. Volunteer! (animal shelter, hospital, food kitchen, nursing home, babysit for a single mom)

YOUR HEALTH AFFIRMATION

"You are what you think about all day long".

– Dr. Robert Schuler

Affirmations are positive statements that describe a situation that you want to see happen. They need to be repeated several times each day with attention and conviction. Your subconscious mind accepts as true the things you keep telling yourself! You will look for and create the situation that you want to bring about. For example, if you keep saying to yourself all day, "I am positive and happy today", you will go through your day actively seeking things to be positive and happy about!

"The mind is everything.
What you think, you become."

-Buddha

Please read your new health affirmation below:

From this day forward, I am designing a life that I love.
I am making healthy choices that love, honor and respect my body.
Every day I am making decisions to feel better and look better.
I am in control of my thoughts, actions, feelings and choices.
I am happier and healthier.

Say this affirmation out loud a few times. **Write it down and put it where you will see it daily.** Write it on several note cards or post it notes. **Bombard your surroundings with it!** Put one on your bathroom mirror, the fridge, desk, everywhere!

"Change your thoughts and you change your world."

-Norman Vincent Peale

Memorize it. Read your affirmation several times each day. Say it out loud. Repeating your affirmation often will leave an imprint on your subconscious mind. Your circumstances will not change until your thoughts change. Think about it when you are making decisions that affect your health and wellness.

Begin to think of the consequences of your choices. For example, when you want a snack, focus on the consequence of the choice of snack. For example, if you choose a candy bar and a soda, you'll experience an energy boost for 20 minutes followed by a CRASH. If you choose cheese, trail mix and an apple with a glass of water, you'll be full, satisfied, and energetic. Make more conscious, deliberate healthy choices and healthy thoughts.

"You become what you think about".

-Earl Nightingale

You will attract what you focus on and think about. Creating new beliefs begins with repetition of thought. Your attitudes and beliefs will positively change your emotions. They will seep into your consciousness.

"Change what you believe and your world changes".

-Francesco Garri Garripoli

I challenge you to choose 2 or 3 more affirmations specific to your life. Look up affirmations and read about them and choose a few that would be meaningful to you. Begin with the general health affirmation suggested and then add a few more to your life as well when you are ready!

A few examples of affirmations:

- I am choosing to focus on the good things about my day.
- I am practicing deep breathing and remaining calm.
- I forgive myself and others for all wrong-doing.
- I am filled with happiness and gratitude.
- I am becoming stronger, slimmer and healthier.
- I am excited about today.
- I am responsible for my thoughts, my beliefs, and my actions.
- I choose to see the best in other people.
- I choose to make positive and healthy choices.

- I am leaving my past behind.
- I am proud of who I am and who I am becoming.
- I am calm and relaxed.
- Happiness is a choice. I choose to be happy.

Keep the same affirmations for about 4 weeks. Then move on to new affirmations. Look for the good in each day.

"I know for sure that what we dwell on is who we become."

- Oprah Winfrey

TAKE THE LIFE SATISFACTION SURVEY BELOW

Assign a numeric value (1-10) to each of the topics listed

Extreme Dissatisfaction   Average   Extreme Satisfaction

1   2   3   4   5   6   7   8   9   10

General Health ___	Home Environment ___
Nutritious Diet ___	Energy Level ___
Adequate Exercise ___	Hair/Skin ___
Finances ___	Body Shape/Weight ___
Spirituality ___	Posture/Breathing ___
Confidence ___	Mood/Emotions ___
Motivation ___	Communication Skills ___
Social Life ___	Cravings (Sugar, Caffeine) ___
Friendships ___	Addictions ___
Relationships ___	Quality Sleep ___
Support System ___	Stress Management ___
Education ___	Relaxation/Fun ___
Career ___	Delegating/Boundaries ___
Home Cooking ___	Life Plans & Goals ___

How to Utilize the Life Satisfaction Survey:

1. Highlight the topics above that you gave a score of 5 or less to.

2. Identify 3 of those highlighted topics that you feel are most important for you to focus on at this point in your life. List them:

   A. _____ B. _____ C. _____

3. Now that you've identified the 3 topics that you want to work on, develop an action plan to begin making changes and improvements. Focus on these three things and begin today to make changes.

GOAL SETTING

"A goal is a dream with a deadline."

-Napoleon Hill

I used to feel kind of like a pin cushion. I pretty much just let life happen to me and I reacted to the punches. As a single mother of 3 busy children, I lived my life so overwhelmed, overcommitted and exhausted that I didn't give much time, attention and thought to my day to day life. I wish I had known more about how to design, create and plan my life to live less of a chaotic existence. I wish I'd focused more on my health and sanity. I wish I'd known more about creating healthy wonderful habits for my children.

We give more thought to planning a trip than we do planning a life! Would you leave your home and set out on a trip to Florida without some prior planning and arrangements? No! You would have saved up the money for the trip, decided if you were driving or flying, and had a hotel room reserved. Your probably even decided on some attractions you were going to go see or activities you were going to do when you got there.

Most of us don't give that much thought to our day to day lives, in terms of planning it and having an end goal. If we don't know where we are going, then how in the world will we get there? We can't live a happy and fulfilling life if we don't identify exactly what it is we'd like to have in our life!

"You are never too old to set another goal or dream a new dream."

-C.S. Lewis

Knowledge is power. I hope to give you some of the tools that I learned the hard way so that your life will be more streamlined and you will do things easier and more efficiently than I did. I want to encourage you to set life goals. I want to help you to be more in control of your life and your destiny. Be the designer and creator of your life. Make it as happy and secure and fun and fantastic as possible. Take some time to identify exactly what it is you want out of life.

Set goals and reward yourself for reaching them! Set both short- term and long -term goals. Also, set both personal and professional goals. See some examples below:

Examples of short-term goals are:

- losing 10 pounds
- completing a graduate class
- volunteering 30 hours for your favorite organization
- building up to run/walk a mile in less than 14 minutes

Examples of rewards for those short-term goals:
- buy a new outfit
- have a spa day
- have a night out with friends
- buy a new piece of jewelry

Some long-term goals might be:
- complete a degree or certification
- make it to your goal weight
- make a career change
- walk or run your first 5k

Examples of rewards for those long-term goals:
- taking a trip
- buying a new wardrobe for your new body size
- buy a new NICE piece of jewelry or a newer car

Setting a reward is important. It will provide a shot of motivation.

The secret of making dreams come true can be summarized in four C's. They are Curiosity, Confidence, Courage, and Constancy; and the greatest of these is Confidence."

-Walt Disney

Let's talk about goal setting in general and how to set a good, realistic goal.

Write down your goals and desires! It is important to get it down on paper. Goals that are not written down are just wishes. Writing it down makes it more real and attainable. It helps to visualize the goal. It paints a picture of what you want. It helps to visually see your goal. For example, if you want to lose 20 pounds and be the size that you were 10 years ago, put a picture of yourself from 10 years ago, on the refrigerator! Surround yourself with reminders.

Be realistic. Set small, attainable goals to ensure success. For example, don't focus on the 20 -pound weight loss, focus on losing 1 or 2 each week. Celebrate those weekly weight loss goals. Make your goal crystal clear. Give your goal a timeline and a deadline.

Be specific. You should be able to measure each goal to see success.

For example, if you want to save $2000 for a trip, instead of thinking about the entire $2000, think in small steps. I can save $40 each week, and in a year, I will have the $2000 and will reward myself with the trip! Celebrate the small steps.

Know what you want. Have the desire and determination to make it happen. Believe that you will achieve it. Be willing to put the work in. Devise a plan with action steps and use concentrated effort toward reaching that goal.

Do something every single day. Feel it. Imagine it. Visualize it. You must want it badly. Be positive and have enthusiasm. It should inspire you. Occasionally, evaluate it and re-focus if necessary.

Allow for setbacks. Don't beat yourself up when you "fall off the wagon" in terms of your goals. You will have a bad day or a setback occasionally. No big deal! You are human. Just begin again the next day with renewed commitment.

Get help! Share your goal with a friend and when possible, seek their assistance and get motivation from them. Seek out resources that make achieving your goal easier for you.

Stop comparing yourself to others. Be happy with yourself. Set goals and reach for dreams that will make you happy. Design a life that is fulfilling and satisfying to you.

Reward yourself for your accomplishments. Celebrate your success! Do something meaningful to you and celebrate!   (get a massage, go to a movie, or buy new jewelry)

A visual representation of your goal is very powerful. For example, if you have a weight loss goal of losing 10 pounds, you could have two glass containers on your kitchen counter. One container would have 10 marbles or rocks in it. Label this container, "pounds to lose". The other container would be labeled "pounds lost". As you lose a pound, you would move the marble. Give something like this a try.

Persistence is the key to reaching your goals.

Know what you want and do something daily toward achieving it.

"When you can taste, smell, and touch your dream, you can enroll the world."

-Jonathan Lockwood Huie

"Fall seven times, stand up eight."

Japanese Proverb

"The difference between try and triumph is just a little umph!"

-Marvin Phillips

"The greatest glory in living lies not in never falling, but in rising every time we fall."

-Nelson Mandela

"Life is either a daring adventure or nothing. Security is mostly a superstition. It does not exist in nature."

-Helen Keller

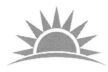

CHAPTER 1: RECAP

The objective of this chapter was to motivate and encourage you to make a commitment to enhance your health and wellness. To truly do this, you must have the **desire** to do so. Next, you need to make a **commitment to yourself.**

Planning, Preparation and Goal-Setting are the key to your success. You wouldn't go on a trip without a roadmap! I will give you the plan and the roadmap. You be the driver…. I'll be your tour guide.

I have provided **Tips for Success** for you. Please re-read your new **10 Commandments for Health** and your new **Health Affirmation**. Review your **Life Satisfaction Survey** and focus on the 3 things you want to improve at this point in your life.

To be successful in making lifestyle changes for health, be very specific and concrete in your intentions and goals. Life each day with purpose and conviction to make healthy choices.

Read on to Chapter 2. Read one section daily and incorporate the information and suggested guidelines into your life. One day at a time, you will create wonderful, new healthy lifestyle habits.

You can do this. Find 20 minutes a day to yourself to read each new segment. Some are longer than others. Some require more thought and planning to incorporate the new suggestions into your life.

By the end of Chapter 7, you will have incorporated many new habits and you will have gained many tips and tools to be the healthiest and happiest you have ever been.

List some things that you intend to start doing.

_____   _____
_____   _____
_____   _____
_____   _____
_____   _____

List some things that you are going to stop doing.

_____   _____
_____   _____
_____   _____

_____   _____
_____   _____

Identify any roadblocks that you have. What can you do about them? _____

_____
_____
_____
_____
_____
_____
_____

Come up with a plan or solution to your roadblocks. _____

_____
_____
_____
_____
_____
_____
_____

CHAPTER 2 - WEEK 1

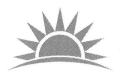

DAY 1: SET YOUR KITCHEN UP FOR SUCCESS

We are going to begin on this very first day by learning the toxic items that you need to eliminate from your kitchen.

As you read the suggestions given, think about making the transition to replace these items with the healthier versions that will be explained in Day Two. You may be able to trash these items completely or give them away. Or, it may make more sense to you to simply use up what you have in your kitchen right now and as you do need to purchase them, make the transition to better quality products at that time.

This is crucial: You must have quality foods to choose from in your home. With every bite of food that you put into your body, you are choosing the quality of your health. Your food "speaks" to your DNA…literally. You are choosing the fuel that goes into your body. You need it to provide the nutrients that **create healthy cells, tissues and organs.** You need to provide the power to your body to develop a **super strong immune system.**

Eliminate:

1. **Eliminate White Products** (sugar, flour, bread, pasta, rice, potatoes, cereal, pastries, cookies, cake). These are "empty calorie" foods with little or no nutritional benefit. These white products turn into sugar when consumed.

2. **Eliminate Unhealthy Oils:** vegetable oil and margarine are examples of items to eliminate! Healthier oils will be explained in day two.

3. **Read labels:** Don't use any products that use these words in their ingredient list: *denatured, refined, hydrogenated, bleached, enriched, trans fats, high fructose corn syrup.*

4. **Eliminate processed foods.** Eliminate foods in a box, instant foods and most fast food. Think about it…if a food could sit in a box for years and you could still consume it, should you? Look at the ingredient list on any meal that comes in a box on a shelf at your grocery store. It will be a long list of items, most of which you cannot pronounce and you have no idea what they are. Don't eat it!

5. **Eliminate artificial ingredients** as much as possible: chemicals, preservatives, pesticides, genetically modified foods (GMO's) artificial colorings, artificial sweeteners, HFCS, MSG, trans fats, nitrates, hormones and antibiotics in food.

6. **Eliminate Traditional Dairy.** This will be explained in more detail later. For now, switch to non-dairy ORGANIC options such as coconut, almond, soy, hemp, cashew, rice products. If you do continue buying regular milk, be sure it is organic.

7. **Eliminate soda of any kind.** Your goal will be to not drink any calories. "Diet" soda is also bad for you though. Even though it has little or no calories, you are setting yourself up for failure by drinking it. The brain recognizes the artificial sweetener as SUGAR, but when the sugar never comes, your body will crave carbs and sugar.

DAY 2:
NEW KITCHEN BASICS!

I want you to learn the Healthy Kitchen Staples that you need to have in your home.

Begin to Focus on the <u>quality</u> of the foods that you eat.

Tip 1: As you look at labels, you want limited ingredients. For example, when looking at an organic bag of frozen fruit, the ingredient list might have blueberries, strawberries, and blackberries. This is a great choice. With all foods that you purchase, the fewer ingredients the better. You need to know what the ingredients are. If there are ingredients you can't pronounce and don't recognize as food, don't eat it! To protect itself, your body will store anything it cannot recognize or digest as fat. So, all the artificial toxic preservatives and chemicals in our food are stored in our fat cells!

Tip 2: Food that expires in a week is a good choice. Real, living food will provide your body with nutrients to benefit your body. Quality food will enable your body to provide you with disease prevention and vitality. We want to live a long time and live well.

Tip 3: If your grandparents would not have recognized what you are eating as FOOD, don't eat it.

Note: I'm providing a quick start guide here, so that you will begin right away to make healthier choices at the grocery store. The suggestions below will be explained in further detail in the weeks to come. There is enough information here to get you started on a healthier, cleaner way of eating for now. Below are the items to add.

1. **Whole Wheat Products:** Look for bread, pasta, crackers, noodles, etc. that have the word "whole" listed in the very first ingredient. That way you know it is a good quality product.

2. **Lean Proteins:** Limit red meat to once per week. Focus on lean protein of high quality. Consider how the animal was raised, fed and treated. Free range, cage free, grass fed…these are better options. Whatever hormones and antibiotics an animal is fed, YOU are consuming as well. Turkey, chicken, cold water fish, wild caught salmon, and quality beef are good options.

3. **Vegetables:** Make it a goal to make half your plate vegetables. Every day, eat some vegetables raw and some cooked. Try to eat a variety of colors of vegetables daily.

4. **Fruits:** For fruits and vegetables both, fresh is best, then frozen, then canned. It is best to eat the fruit instead of drinking fruit juice. Your goal is to eat 1 cup of at least 3 different fruits every day early in the day…before mid-day. Then, don't eat any more fruit all day. (1 cup total of mixed fruits daily)

5. **Try ORGANIC Dairy Alternatives** such as almond milk, soy milk, rice milk, cashew milk, coconut milk, or hemp milk. If you do want traditional dairy products, be sure to purchase organic. Dairy is not as healthy as it used to be. Factory farming practices to maximize profits mean that animals are often not fed foods they were meant to eat. They are not out in fields in the sunshine and not allowed to roam freely eating the foods nature meant for them to consume. They become sick. They are given antibiotics, growth hormone, steroids, etc. Anything the animal ingested, we ingest. Therefore, organic dairy or dairy alternatives are the best choice.

6. **Use Healthy Oils** such as extra virgin olive oil, coconut oil, sesame oil, grapeseed oil, canola oil, macadamia nut oil and organic butter.

7. **Drinks** Focus on the goal of not drinking any calories. Stick with coffee, tea and water. Use non-dairy creamer and stevia instead of sugar.

8. **Healthy Sugar Alternatives:** stevia, 100% maple syrup, raw local honey, brown rice syrup, and organic raw agave nectar are good choices.

9. **Make it a goal to eliminate added sugar to your foods.** This is important for energy and weight loss. If you want to be healthy, fit, and lean, eliminate added sugar to your diet.

Why Eat Lean and Clean?

The body can protect, heal itself, and keep you healthy if you give it the building blocks that it needs. When we eat foods that do not contain nutrients and health properties that nourish it, we continue to crave more and more food. Doesn't it seem odd that so many of us are overweight, yet sick and malnourished? To protect your vital organs, any foreign substances that the body can't digest and doesn't know what to do with is stored inside your fat cells. This explains why so many of us are very large around out middle!

Most disease is preventable! As I learned at the Institute for Integrative Nutrition, **Food Is Medicine.** Nutritious food provides medicinal components and properties to your body. By your choice of quality food or junk food you literally are choosing whether you enhance your biological chemistry or destroy it. Eat for vitality and health. Eat healthy to be healthy.

Cravings

Pay attention to the cravings that you have. Do you have any food addictions? Perhaps sugar or caffeine are issues for you. Consider a detox diet or an elimination diet. There are many different types of them. If you focus on getting nutrient dense foods and enough water into your daily meal plan, your body will not crave the unhealthy foods you used to eat. Don't think about what you can't have, focus on getting the right things in your body every day.

Focus on eating real, living food that expires in a week.

Now is the time! There is no perfect time. Begin today. Not next Monday. Not tomorrow. Today! Start adopting new healthy habits so you can be the person you want to be.

"I am not a product of my circumstances.
I am a product of my decisions."

-Stephen Covey

DAY 3:
POWER IN PLANNING & PREPARATION

One of the most important lifestyle habits you can create is simply to learn to take a few minutes each week to plan and prepare for the week. Below are a few tips to get you started!

Tip 1: Take the time to **plan** your meals, snacks and grocery lists. **Preparing** your healthy meals and snacks is vital to your success. I'll make this very simple for you!

Tip 2: **Keep healthy snacks and water with you.** I never leave home without tea or water with me in the car or in my bag. I keep a protein bar or trail mix with me as well. This greatly reduces my likelihood to go through a drive through restaurant for a snack or drink!

Tip 3: Look at your calendar. Carve out two 90 minute blocks of time each week for **food preparation.**

What I do to make this work:

Almost every Sunday of my life I plan meals for the week. I cook two times each week. I usually cook on Sunday and Wednesday. Each time I cook, I prepare 2 protein dishes and 4 vegetable dishes. That way I can mix and match different veggies and proteins together. I usually use quinoa or couscous for a healthy grain. (or I don't have a grain at all).

I do the snack preparation during those same two blocks of time. In baggies, I put different fruits and veggies. For example, in one baggie I might have grapes, blueberries and cherries. In another baggie, I might have carrots, celery and bell peppers. I buy protein bars and protein shakes as well. If you have healthy things ready to grab and have with you, you take away the need and temptation to buy or eat unhealthy foods and snacks. Set yourself up for success by having easy to grab choices.

Why this works: Planning the meals and snacks allows you to be in control. You can manage your healthy eating path when you have things already ready to eat. You will have wonderful choices in front of you when you open the refrigerator door! Organize your refrigerator so that the healthy choices are in front, in plain sight. Put your meals and snacks in single serving containers, ready to go.

Simplicity and Routine: Keep repeating these healthy habits. Set yourself up for success. Soon, this will be second nature to you and you'll feel like you are on auto-pilot. The routine provides stability and new wonderful habits.

Example: On Sunday, I made the following:

Proteins: Chicken and Salmon

Vegetables: Stir fry vegetables, Brussels Sprouts, Carrots, Asparagus

Grain: Quinoa and Kale Blend

I mixed and matched the foods I cooked into these meals for lunches and dinners for 3 days:

Dinner: Chicken, Brussels Sprouts, Quinoa and Kale Blend

Lunch: A bowl with these mixed together: Stir fry Veggies and chicken

Dinner: Salmon, Carrots, Asparagus

Lunch: Salad greens with chicken

Dinner: Stir Fry Veggies with pieces of salmon and Brussels Sprouts

Lunch: A bowl with these things mixed together: Quinoa and Kale Blend and Chicken

Time Saver Tips

So, you see in the previous example, **I cooked once, and this provided 6 meals** in some variety, using those foods I spent 60-90 minutes making. This is a huge time saver. And you are so much more likely to eat healthfully when it is ready and will only take a few minutes to get warmed up. In less time than you would spend sitting and waiting in a drive through window to buy unhealthy "food", you could have quality, delicious food at home.

I bought segmented plates with lids that are perfect for meal preparation. On each plate, I put a protein and 2 vegetable dishes, or a protein, 1 vegetable, and 1 grain. I also use small glass bowls with lids for the lunch combinations.

My dog, Baxter benefits from this as well. Some of the chicken, salmon, fish, or beef I make goes in his dog dish as well. He's a happy boy, that's for sure!

"If you do what you've always done,
you'll get what you've always gotten."

-Tony Robins

Create these habits: (Routine, Simplicity, and Repetition)

- Once a week, sit down and plan your meals and snacks.

- From your list of meals and snacks, make a grocery list. Go to the grocery store when you are NOT hungry and stick to your list.

- I recommend that you set aside two 60 -90 minute blocks of time each week to cook

- While you are cooking, you will also do any snack preparation that you need to do.

- Put your food plan on REPEAT! Keep it simple. Take the time to plan 2 weeks' worth of meals and snacks with corresponding grocery lists. Simply having a rotation of foods that are healthy and that you enjoy will help you to eat healthfully without having to think about it much. It will help you with consistency and take the planning time down to a minimum.

- Supersize the right way! Make one meal a day a salad. You can eat a large volume of food and be full and satisfied.

- Make half of your plate vegetables at every meal.

"Energy and persistence conquer all things."

-Benjamin Franklin

A Sample Weekly Grocery Store List:

4 proteins: cold water fish, wild salmon, organic chicken, grass fed beef

8 vegetables: frozen bag of stir fry, mixed salad greens, carrots, asparagus, spinach, sweet potatoes, broccoli/cauliflower/carrot mix, mixed vegetables

6 fruits: apples, bananas, watermelon, blueberries, grapes, cherries

Grains: whole wheat bread, whole wheat pasta, couscous, oatmeal

Snacks: protein bars, popcorn, baked chips and salsa, trail mix, hummus, carrot sticks, protein drinks, Greek yogurt, celery sticks, almond butter.

Dairy/Dairy Alternative: Cage free eggs, Chocolate Almond Milk, Coconut Milk, Butter

Note: A very comprehensive Grocery Store List will be provided on page 174-175.

My Guilty Pleasure:

100% cocoa is good for you! Try this delicious drink!

Add to a cup of coffee: 1 teaspoon of 100% cocoa, a few drops of stevia and a splash of chocolate almond milk! YUMMY!

DAY 4: MOVE IT!

Today, I want you to focus on incorporating fitness into your lifestyle. Incorporating movement into your life is absolutely necessary to your health. Fitness is a lifestyle, not a fad. It is something you must add into your day. No excuses! Start living a healthier life TODAY!

The minimum amount of exercise your body needs for health is:

- 30 minutes of cardio 5 times each week
- 30 minutes of strength movements each week

This is not that hard to do and there are GREAT BENEFITS to you physically and mentally.

1. Exercising regularly will greatly **reduce risk of disease**. Most disease is preventable!

2. It will also allow you to more gracefully age and have good functional movement as you age. You will want to be able to **live long, but also live well!** You want to be able to care of yourself and your home and not be dependent on others. To keep your independence, you must maintain movement in your life.

3. Exercise releases endorphins which are the **"feel good" hormones.** They are natural chemicals released by the brain that improve your mood, relieve pain, reduce stress, and produce "well-being". The best way to release endorphins is to exercise!

4. You'll feel more energetic and confident.

5. You'll look better!

6. You'll start to fit back into that 70% of clothes in your closet that are too tight!

7. Exercise is a natural stress reducer.

"If there is no struggle, there is no progress."

-Frederick Douglass

Real Life Story:

In my younger years, I ran 5 or 6 miles on most days. I experienced that "runners high" and was an absolute bear if I didn't get my "fix". It really does do the mind and body a world of good to exercise. Truthfully though, now in my late 50's I realize how much wear and tear the body experiences from running on pavement. Knowing what I now know, I would have limited the running on the streets!

I hope I've convinced you to make movement a part of your daily lifestyle plan! Choose exercises or movements that you enjoy. Vary the type of exercise. Make it happen! Reach you better body goals! It doesn't matter HOW you move, just that you move!

Tips:

1. Decide on an **exercise plan**. Think about what you enjoy doing and when you can fit it into your busy week.

2. Make it a priority. **Schedule it!** Put it on your calendar and keep this appointment for yourself. It is a must.

3. Make yourself a promise to incorporate a two-day rule! Never let more than two days go by without at least a 30-minute fitness segment.

4. It helps to enlist a friend to exercise with you. An **exercise buddy** will make you both more accountable to show up!

5. Consider hiring a **personal trainer** to teach you some strength and cardio movements. To make it less expensive, seek out a small group personal training program or class. The cost will be reduced greatly in a small group setting. Once you meet with a trainer several times, you will know a lot more to do on your own and have a skill set of exercises and movements to choose from.

6. If you enjoy **classes**, join a gym or fitness club that offers a variety of classes. Mix it up! Take a strength class 2 days a week, and a variety of cardio classes on 3 days a week. A great mix would be to take a water aerobics class a day or two and land aerobics classes a day or two a week.

7. **Motivation:** Treat yourself to new fitness clothes and shoes. When you look good, you FEEL good!

8. **Find music that inspires you!** Develop a fitness playlist!

Cardio Ideas:

1. If you are not currently exercising, **start with walking.** Weather permitting, simply walk out your door, walk 15 minutes away from your home and turn around and walk back. Over time, you can increase the pace or increase the distance or both. For now, simply begin with a moderate walk. If weather is bad, find an indoor place such as a mall to walk in out of the weather. Another idea is to find a DVD walking program or other fitness activity you can do in your home.

2. **Any exercise machine** (treadmill, climber, bicycle, elliptical, etc.) is great for your cardio workout. Remember, your goal is 30 minutes, but that may be too difficult to do if you are just beginning! If so, begin with 15 minutes and increase by 5 minutes each week or every other week until you are at the 30 -minute goal.

Strength Training Ideas:
(use equipment or your own body weight!)

1. You can get your 30 minutes each week in very easily. Ideally you want to split the strength training time up into **2 segments** of 15 minutes. (or 3 segments of 10 minutes)

2. Examples of **body weight strength training** are sports yoga, Pilates moves, or any activity where you are using your own body strength such as push -ups against a wall or on the floor, mountain climbers or burpees.

3. Various **equipment** can be used for strength and toning: 2 full water bottles, any hand weights, exercise band, barbell, kettle ball, medicine ball, etc.

4. Learn exercises for the basics muscle groups: biceps, triceps, back, shoulders, abs, lower back, core, hips, and legs. This is an example of when a trainer would be beneficial. They could teach you the basics or if you are a member of a gym, they can show you how to properly use the weight equipment.

5. If you don't want to go to a gym, there are wonderful fitness DVD's that you can purchase and do at home!

Set Specific Fitness Goals:

It is necessary to sit down once a week and schedule your fitness activities. Look over your work and family obligations and see where it will fit in.

Important: You must be specific when you set your fitness goals:

What?   (Zumba class, water aerobics, walk, jog, treadmill, bike, weights)

Where?   (park, gym, your home, pool)

When?   (when you first wake up, 5:00, right after work)

How?   (using target heart rate, using perceived exertion, moderate, high intensity)

How long?   (30 minutes, 1 hour, 40 minutes, 15 minutes)

How far?   (1 mile, 3 miles)

Who?   (other class members, friend, kids, co-worker)

Sample week of fitness goals:

Monday	4:30 -5:30	Cardio Class followed by 15- minute upper body workout.
Tuesday	6:00-6:45	Walk dog in park 1.5 miles, take him home, then walk 1 more mile.
Wednesday	day off	
Thursday	5:30-6:30	Water Aerobics class and then 15 min lower body workout
Friday	6:00-6:45	Walk dog in park 1.5 miles, take him home, then walk 1 more mile.
Saturday	10:00-11:00	Pump RX class (strength class)
Sunday	2:00	Walk the dog 1.5 miles, then walk/jog 30 minutes more.

IS TIME a ROADBLOCK?

Try an Express Workout!

CHUNKS OF TIME will work!

If you truly do not have time to do a 30-minute cardio segment:

- Do 10 minutes of cardio 3 times during the day
- Do 15 minutes of cardio two times during the day
- For every hour that you sit, get up and move for 10 minutes
- Take the steps instead of the elevator
- Park further away from the doors at work or when shopping
- If possible, walk or bike to work or when doing errands
- Plan activities that involve fitness with your friends and family

Other factors to consider in planning your workout: Intensity, Time, and Distance

Exercise Intensity means how hard you are working during your workout. You may want to use a scale of **perceived exertion.** On this scale, a 1 is sitting on the couch. A 10 would be a full out run at your fastest speed. You want to exercise at a 6, 7, or 8 on this scale. A good rule of thumb is that you should be able to talk during exercise. If you are unable to talk a little during exercise, you are probably working too hard!

You can choose to use **"time" or "distance"** as you plan your fitness activity. For example, you can decide to walk for 30 minutes. Or, you could choose to walk two miles.

One effective way to exercise is to try to stay in your **target heart rate zone** during exercise. Go to sparkpeople.com or webmd.com to see a chart or calculate your training zone if you want to use this method. It is based on your age. You want your heart rate to stay in a range of 65% to 85% of your maximum heart rate.

DAY 5: LOG IT!

You have learned the fitness basics. Today, you need to decide on a method of logging your fitness activity.

Starting today, begin by simply getting a calendar and write down your fitness activity. Keep it where you see it daily. The side of the refrigerator is a good place. Don't ever let more than 2 days is a row go by without exercising. If you don't make yourself write it down and have that visual reminder, you'll tend to feel like you exercise more than you do.

Start this new healthy habit today!

Are you a "techy"?

You might be more comfortable using an app on your phone or computer to keep a record of your fitness activity. Either way is fine. Use the method that is easiest for you.

There are many apps to use for fitness tracking. Below are a few for you to check out. Any of them are great. Find one that you like!

- MyFitnessPal
- Lose it!
- Noom Coach
- HAPIcoach

Remember your goal is:

- Cardio 30 minutes 5 days per week
- Strength 30 minutes per week

Which type of "logging" method will you use to keep track of your fitness activity?
Begin today!

DAY 6: HYDRATE FOR HEALTH

Starting today, make a commitment to drink enough water!
It is so important for health and healing!

Water is the most important nutrient of all! **Water makes up 60% of our body and 50% of our blood.** When we do not drink enough water, we may experience the following: headaches, fatigue, hunger, or sugar cravings. Your health is dependent on the quantity and quality of the water that you drink. Many symptoms of disease would go away, if we drank enough water. It provides energy for breathing, growth, maintenance, immunity, and detoxification.

Dehydration is often mistaken for hunger. Keep pure, filtered water with you always.

How much water do YOU need to drink each day? A good goal is to divide your body weight in half and drink that number of ounces per day. For example, a person who weighs 160 pounds should consume at least 80 ounces of water. Figure out what that is for you.

Suggestion: Buy a nice insulated water bottle and figure out how many ounces it holds and how many times you need to fill it up daily. Start today to get enough water in. You will feel amazing! Carry this water bottle with you everywhere!

Functions of water: Water helps convert food into energy. It helps regulate body temperature, carries nutrients, minerals, proteins, and carbohydrates, it lubricates joints, and it cleanses the body and excretes wastes through urine.

Just as you are what you eat, you are what you drink as well!

Tricks to make yourself drink more WATER!!

- Put frozen berries in ice cube trays. Put them in your glass of water. It will flavor the water and make it more enjoyable. You can also add these to tea.

- Add just a splash of 100% juice to your plain or sparkling water.

- Add a few drops of cinnamon extract or sea salt to your water. (quality sea salt is not white! It is beige or pink)

- Drink coconut water.

- Keep a pitcher of water in the fridge with slices of any fruit. (oranges, kiwi, lemon, lime, cucumber, etc.) It needs to sit for several hours to really flavor the water.

- Make yourself alternate water with other beverages. I won't allow myself to drink tea or coffee until I have had a water.

- Drink a large glass of water about 20 minutes before meals. Do the same thing when you are craving a snack. Wait that 20-minute period and see you even still want the snack. Many times, you are dehydrated, and you just know you are craving something. A lot of times, just the water will satisfy you!

- **Consume foods with high water content!** Leafy greens, melons, tomatoes, eggplant, squash, cucumbers, lemons, radishes, strawberries, celery, iceberg lettuce, zucchini, apricot, blueberry, oranges, peaches, pineapple, plums, raspberries.

This works for my daughter, Megan! Give it a try.

My daughter, Megan, takes a gallon jug of water to work with her every morning. Her rule is she can't leave work until it is empty. She is a teacher. What a great example she is setting for her students. She allows her students to bring water into her classroom as well.

Making a commitment to drink plenty of water has been instrumental in Megan's recent weight loss journey. She also noticed a great side effect. She has had less headaches and sinus problems. She's also getting some exercise in her day, sprinting to the restroom between all those class changes.

DAY 7:
GO FOR GREENS

Your new healthy habit for today is to focus on getting in enough GREEN foods. Most people do not eat nearly enough.

A few of the reasons why GREENS are so important:

- Blood purification
- Cancer prevention
- Strengthen immune system
- Improve lung, kidney, gall bladder and kidney function

Tip: Every day try to eat some raw and some cooked! You'll get different health benefits by including both in your diet. Make a new habit of eating raw veggies before dinner.

Foods to include in your weekly meal planning:

Broccoli	Bok Choy	Napa Cabbage	Kale
Collard Greens	Watercress	Mustard Greens	Dandelion
Green Cabbage	Arugula	Endive	Chicory
Lettuce	Spinach	Swiss Chard	Parsley

Real Life Story:

I started a new healthy habit that you might incorporate into your life too! Every time I cook, I get out a small plate with raw veggies. Usually broccoli, carrots, peppers and cauliflower. I put a little yogurt based ranch out with it. I eat the veggies while I'm doing food prep. I also drink a glass of water. Then, when it comes to meal time, I don't overeat, because I'm not as "starved" as I would have been if I hadn't snacked on this healthy appetizer!

Remember, GO GREEN for a healthy immune system and Disease Prevention

Super Green Powdered Mixes: There are many brands of power greens. These powdered green mixes contain wonderful healthy powerhouses that we would not normally get in our diet. Sea vegetables, wheat grasses, and many more wonderful health boosting properties are in these green mixes. I encourage you to get some and incorporate it into your lifestyle. You can put it in smoothies, stir fry, or soups. You will never know it's in there and your body will benefit from it greatly.

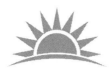

CHAPTER 2: RECAP

Each day this week you have focused on a different aspect of health. Your goal is to incorporate as many suggestions and lifestyle changes into your lifestyle.

1. Over time continue with your **Kitchen Clean Up!** As you need to replace items, purchase healthier versions. For example, replace sugar with stevia and replace white bread with whole wheat bread.

2. Also, over time, continue to purchase new **Quality Kitchen Basics**.

3. Remember there is **Power in Planning and Preparation**. You must take the time to plan your meals and prepare proteins, vegetables, and snacks. Routine and repetition are good. Keep it simple.

4. Review the fitness basics. You must **add movement into your lifestyle.** Sit down and plan your fitness schedule. Put it on your calendar!

5. **Log it!** You must keep track of your fitness activity. A visual is important. Use a calendar page or an app for this!

6. Drinking enough water is essential. **Hydrate for Health!** Hydration Heals! If we all just drank enough water, we'd have less sinus headaches and less health issues!

7. Your new motto this week is, **"GO FOR GREENS".** Get more greens into your day. Make it a goal to eat some raw and some steamed each day.

List some things that you intend to start doing.

_____   _____
_____   _____
_____   _____
_____   _____
_____   _____

List some things that you are going to stop doing.

_____ _____

_____ _____

_____ _____

_____ _____

_____ _____

Identify any roadblocks that you have. What can you do about them? _____

_____

_____

_____

_____

_____

Come up with a plan or solution to your roadblocks. _____

_____

_____

_____

_____

_____

CHAPTER 3 - WEEK 2

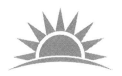

DAY 1: LEAN PROTEIN POWER

Protein plays a huge role in your life!

Protein is good for you. It helps keep your energy up and helps you to feel full and satisfied. But be careful! The excess protein that you consume is stored as fat! There are many other health issue concerns with consumption of too much protein: it may lead to kidney disease, cancers, osteoporosis or kidney stones. The quality of the protein is important. Other considerations are the type of protein and the amount of protein you consume.

Protein is found in bone, muscle, hemoglobin, myoglobin, hormones, antibodies and enzymes. It makes up almost half of your body!

- Protein is responsible for the building of and repair of body tissues.
- Protein produces hormones, enzymes and other substances the body needs.
- It regulates body process, such as transportation of nutrients, water balancing and contraction of muscles.
- Protein keeps the body healthy by resisting disease.
- It prevents us from becoming fatigued by producing stamina and energy.

How much protein do you need? Most of us eat too much protein! Your plan for protein is to eat a small amount (3 to 4 ounces) of lean protein several times through the day (3- 5 times during the day). If you work out more than 30 minutes a day, you want to add a little more protein to your food plan.

Animal protein sources: The best sources are ones that are complete proteins. These contain all the essential amino acids: beef, chicken, fish, eggs, milk, and other products from animal sources. (Be sure to purchase grass fed, free range, organic products that are free of hormones, antibiotics, growth hormones). Better cuts of meat are USDA Prime or Choice.

Beware of Nitrates: Be sure to purchase nitrate free, uncured meats that the body can digest safely. Look at the labels. Most packaged meats and lunch meats contain nitrates. They are devastating to the body. Avoid canned soups with meat in them. Imagine the preservatives needed! It's so easy to make fresh stew, chili, or soup in the crock pot or on top of the stove. Go for that instead.

Make it your goal to eat more vegetarian sources of protein. These are powerful for your health and excellent protein sources: grains, beans (black beans, chickpeas, pinto beans, lima beans, black-eyed peas, edamame, soy beans), green leafy vegetables, broccoli, lentils, tofu, corn tortillas, nuts, seeds, soymilk, fortified juices, tofu, veggie burger, soymilk and soy yogurt.

Great grains: Whole grains are an excellent source of nutrition (enzymes, iron, dietary fiber, Vitamin E and B complex vitamins). Because the body absorbs grains slowly, they provide sustained and high-quality energy. Quinoa, brown rice, buckwheat, oats, amaranth, barley, bulgur, cornmeal, couscous, kamut, millet, rye, wild rice, oats, brown whole wheat pasta and whole grain breads are good sources.

Good legumes: beans, lentils, peas, peanuts, traditional soy products

Protein Powders: Good sources are whey or pea. Look for 14-21 grams of protein per serving and 5 grams or lower in sugar.

Protein Bars: These can be GREAT or HORRIBLE for you. Just look at the label for the following information and choose a nutritious kind of protein bar.

Look for a protein bar that has at least 4 of the 5 criteria below:

- **Protein** – at least 10 grams or more
- **Sugar** – no more than 16 grams of sugar. The sugar should be from real fruit, not added sugars
- **Calories** – especially if this is a snack and not a meal replacement, try to stick to 350 calories or lower
- **Fat** – 5 grams of fat or lower and zero trans fats
- **Fiber** – to help you feel full and satisfied, 5 grams or more of fiber should be in the bar. If weight loss is your focus, look for high fiber bars.

DAY 2:
HEALTHY FATS ARE WHERE IT'S AT!

The lesson for you to learn today is about what fats to include in your diet and which ones to eliminate! I also want you to realize that the right fats are important to include in your diet!

One common mistake people make when trying to lose weight is that they go on a no fat or low fat diet. Dietary fat is an important energy source for the body. Many important body functions cannot be performed correctly without the healthy fats.

Fats are necessary in the diet!

- Fats assist with **regulation** of your blood pressure, heart rate, blood vessel constriction, blood clotting, hormone regulation and various nervous system functions.

- **Your brain is largely made up of fats!**

- **Cellular regeneration** relies on healthy fats.

- For your body to **BURN fat** and function properly, you must supply it with necessary healthy fats!

- Healthy fats **reduce inflammation** in the body

- They help **lower the "bad"** LDL cholesterol

Not all fats are created equal however!
Let's focus on the good fats!

MUFA's are good fats! MUFA is short for monounsaturated fats. They remain liquid at room temperature, but may solidify in the refrigerator.

Polyunsaturated Fats are also good fats. They remain in liquid form both at room temperature and in the refrigerator.

Good sources of MUFA's and Polyunsaturated Fats are:

- Healthy Oils (extra virgin olive, coconut, sesame, canola, red palm, macadamia nut, safflower, grapeseed, sunflower, soybean, peanut, flaxseed, ghee, organic butter)

- Olives

- Nuts (cashews, walnuts, pecans, almonds, pistachio, hazelnut, brazil)

- Seeds (flax, chia, pumpkin, hemp, sunflower, sesame)

- Avocado

- Dark Chocolate (70% cacao and higher)

- Nut Butters: Peanut butter, almond butter, cashew butter

Make the healthy fats part of your daily food intake! They keep your brain healthy, extend your life, target body fat, and help build a strong immune system!

More sources of healthy fats are:

- Fish (trout, herring, mackerel, sardines)

- Wild caught tuna or salmon
- Organic eggs
- Organic hard cheeses such as Mozzarella or Cheddar
- High quality meats (grass fed, free range)
- Green foods
- Traditional Organic Soy Products

Important Tip: If you do not eat fish, salmon or other omega 3 rich foods on a routine basis, consider a supplement! There are many good products to choose from. A few of them are krill oil, cod liver oil, and omega 3 swirl.

Traditional Soy Products are good for you! Try to incorporate these into your food plan: Miso, soy beans, yogurt, kefir, kimchee, tempeh, kombucha, natto, Worcestershire, soy sauce, sauerkraut, refrigerated pickles, sour cream.

What FATS do you need to ELIMINATE or at least greatly LIMIT?
SAY NO TO: Saturated Fats, Trans Fats or Hydrogenated Fats

Saturated fats are the main cause of high blood pressure. Most saturated fats come from animals and animal products. Saturated fats become solid or semi-solid at room temperature.

Animal sources of saturated fat include: beef, veal, lamb, pork, lard, poultry, butter, cream, milk, cheese, dairy products made from whole or 2 percent milk. Marbling in red meat and sticks of butter are prime examples.

Plant Sources of saturated fat: coconut, coconut oil, palm oil and palm kernel oil and cocoa butter.

Trans Fats (TFA) or Hydrogenated Fats also raise blood cholesterol. These types of fats are bad news! They increase inflammation, spike insulin levels and increase triglyceride levels. Unfortunately, these particular fats are cheap and effective for manufacturers. They make our food taste crispier and more delicious. Trans fats are found in nearly every food that contains shortening.

Trans Fats Raise your BAD Cholesterol (LDL) and lower your good cholesterol (HDL).

Look at the labels on the foods your purchase. Look for the words, "hydrogenated" or partially hydrogenated" and **avoid** them! Purchase products that state "0 trans- fat". Also, limit fried foods.

Tips for Oils:

- Don't purchase "denatured, bleached, or hydrogenated" oils.
- Do purchase cold pressed and / or unrefined oils.
- Do store in dark bottles, away from sunlight and heat
- To flavor foods (not for baking) use walnut oil, butter, or coconut butter.
- If you haven't before, bake with macadamia nut oil.
- Use toasted sesame oil for stir fry.
- Use parchment paper for baking (up to 450 degrees) and use much less oil!
- Drizzle the oil on the food that you are cooking, instead of in the pan.

DAY 3:
COMPLEX SMART CARBS

Today's lesson is about which carbohydrates are good for you.

Basically, a good carb is a fruit or vegetable. Some are better than others, but all fruits and vegetables in their natural raw state the way that God made them are good for you.

Carbohydrates provide energy to the cells in our body. They fuel the basal metabolic rate and activity levels. They play an important role in the immune system, in reproduction, and assist with blood clotting. They are needed for optimum health and provide nutrients necessary for good brain function.

Good Carbs:

Good Carbs provide your body with energy, optimum nutrition, brain and organ function and a healthy, pleasing appearance! They will help with weight loss, lowering cholesterol, prevent constipation, reduce tri-glycerides, carry toxins out of the body, help avoid diabetes, maintain stable blood sugar (providing consistent sustained energy rather than the high/low rollercoaster of blood sugar levels), and decrease risk of heart disease.

Good Carb List: Think of foods from nature that are in their raw state. Without additives and preservatives and processing, food is healthier. Raw or steamed vegetables, fruits, legumes, beans, nuts and seeds are "good carbs". High fiber 100% whole grain products, and most organic dairy are good sources as well. Foods with resistant starches are especially good. They are digested slowly and help your blood sugar to remain stable. Include these in your meals: rolled oats, banana, beans, peas, potatoes that are cooled, and artichoke.

Bad Carbs:

Bad carbs are detrimental to a healthy diet. Consuming a lot of these will rapidly **sabotage your health** and weight management goals. **Bad carbs are foods that have been highly refined and processed.** This removes most of the healthy fiber and the nutritional value! They are loaded with high-calorie fats, sweeteners, preservatives and other unhealthy additives. Although they are very tasty, they cause a dramatic spike of insulin in the body. This overworks your pancreas and causes your body to store the excess fat. Consuming too many "bad carbs" will lead to diabetes, heart disease, obesity, Alzheimer's, arthritis, and stroke.

Bad Carb List: jelly, jams, candies, sodas, fruit drinks and juices, pudding, processed refined grains like white rice, white potatoes, all white bread and pasta made with any refined flour, cakes, cookies, and bakery products.

It it's white, don't take a bite! Unless it's cauliflower!

Fiber:

Fiber is the part of the plant that your body can't absorb or digest

Fiber is carbohydrate that is indigestible. Most Americans do not get enough fiber in their diet. Soluble fiber is in foods such as citrus fruit, prunes, beans, barley, legumes, rye, nuts and seeds, vegetables, oats, brown rice, wheat bran and whole grains.

This insoluble fiber helps with digestion. It delays stomach emptying and slows absorption. This will put blood sugar into the body slower (great for diabetics).

The benefits of fiber: (make it your goal to eat at least 25 grams daily)

- Improves cholesterol
- Helps maintain a healthy weight
- Decreases disease risk
- Helps you feel full and satisfied
- Helps regulate the digestive tract
- Aids and slows digestion

Beans and Fiber are a dieter's best friend!

Beans make you feel full. They increase fat burning and have anti-inflammatory properties. Good sources are kidney, navy, pinto, black, chickpea, and butter beans. Others include fat free refried and instant bean soups.

Make it your goal to fill up half of your plate with vegetables at every meal.
You will be full, happy, satisfied and healthy.

DAY 4:
STRENGTH AND TONE ZONE

Today I want you to really buy in to why you need to add strength training to your fitness routine. There are so many benefits to toning and strengthening our bodies!

As we age, our metabolism slows down. To fight that, we need to do strength training. As you gain lean muscle, your metabolism will increase. This metabolism boost is 24 hours a day, 7 days a week!

One pound of fat burns about 3 calories a day. A pound of muscle burns about 50 calories a day! So, the more muscle you build, the faster your metabolism is all the time. So, strength training will help with your battle to budge the pudge!

By toning and strengthening, your body will burn more calories even when it is at rest!

Here are some facts about strength training:

- It keeps muscles and bones strong
- It allows your body to burn more calories at rest (increases metabolism)
- Strength training is anti-aging
- It keeps joints healthy and helps prevent bone loss

Strength Training is so easy to do and is NOT time consuming. As mentioned earlier, you just need to do strength training 30 minutes each week. So, this could be two 15 minute segments or three 10 minute segments.

Use a variety of methods in your strength training. That way you will get benefits of each type of activity. Some suggestions:

- Body weight exercises: planks, push-ups, burpees, mountain climbers, yoga, Pilates
- Barbell or weighted bar
- Hand weights, kettlebell or fitness bands

Tips for Using Weights:

1. Start with a lighter weight and work on your form. Begin with doing one set of 12 repetitions. Once this feels easy, move to 2 sets. Then add a third set of 12. Once this is easy, use a slightly heavier weight and begin the process again.

2. Another option is to use a weight that is more challenging to you and do one set of 15 repetitions. Use a heavy enough weight that it is doable but challenging to finish that 15th repetition.

3. There are wonderful DVD's out there for strength training. Purchase one and do your 30 minutes each week. You can find these on on-line or at most store chains.

4. Join a strength and toning type of class or join a gym and use the weight equipment or circuit station area that is available.

DAY 5: GRATITUDE ATTITUDE

Let's take time today to appreciate the things we have and to be grateful for them.

"I was complaining that I had no shoes until I met a man who had no feet."

-Confucius

In my own life, so many times when I've let myself "go there" to the self-pity zone, I've been startled back to reality when I hear about something that another person is going through that is so much worse. I'm sure this happens to you too. Our issue or problem is put back in perspective.

Instead of thinking about what we don't have, focus on what we DO have and be thankful for it. You can't help but be happy if you do this. It is easy to look at the lives of others and envy what they have. We sometimes think that someone else's life looks so easy, calm and wonderful. I have learned that looks can be deceiving. We don't know what anyone else's struggles and issues are. We all have them!

Take the time and energy to enjoy your family and friends. Enjoy your home and surround yourself with things that bring you joy. Concentrate on enjoying what you have and where you are right now.

Life is made of todays, not of tomorrows! Life doesn't have to be perfect to be enjoyed. Don't let the "things" that you want in the future keep you from enjoying the now.

Your life will be so much happier if you enjoy each day and actively LOOK FOR things to be grateful for each day. This goes for the people in your life too. We all have faults. Choose to focus on the good things about your loved ones and less about their faults.

Gratitude Rock: The next time you go shopping, look for a few small, beautiful rocks, marbles or beads. Make these your gratitude reminders. I have them everywhere in my surroundings and every time I see one, it is my visual reminder to focus on something I'm grateful for. I have them in my change purse, in my car, on kitchen windowsill, on my office desk, and in my bathroom. My LARGE gratitude rocks are my Himalayan sea salt lamps. I love them! The one in my office even has a place at the top to put essential oils. Consider getting one for your home!

Begin to keep a gratitude journal.

By my bed, I have a legal pad for journaling. I challenge you to get a notebook or legal pad and keep it by your bed too. Every night before you go to sleep, write down 3 things you are grateful for. As time goes on and you create this new habit, you will begin to go through every day of your life **LOOKING for things to be grateful for.** The shift to positive thinking will make your days more pleasant. Doing this will truly **cultivate a grateful heart.** Give it a try!

"Be thankful for what you have; you'll end up having more. If you concentrate on what you don't have, you will never, ever have enough.

-Oprah Winfrey

DAY 6:
DIVE IN FOR BETTER DIGESTION

Many people have difficulties with digestion. There are many things you can do to aid digestion and limit the issues that you might have.

The first thing I want to mention in terms of digestive issues is gluten.

Do you have gluten sensitivity?

There are many different health issues related to gluten. There are also many varieties of wheat used in food products. Only a very small percentage of the population has celiac disease, but many of us are gluten sensitive.

The **symptoms** of gluten sensitivity are: brain fog, depression, weight gain, headaches, bloating, diarrhea, irritable bowel, skin rash, constipation, or a burning in the stomach after eating. Do you have any of those symptoms?

To find out if gluten is an issue for you: For a 2- week period, eliminate eating grains of any kind; stick to foods that have one ingredient (whole foods). These are vegetables and fruits, meat, fish, dairy, lentils, rice, corn, dairy, high quality chocolate, water, tea, and red wine. For this 2 weeks, completely avoid wheat, rye, and barley to see if your symptoms go away! (There are many "gluten free" products that you can purchase if you don't want to strictly stick to the food list given previously)

Digestive Health Recommendations:

1. Drink a glass of **water** 20 minutes before eating. Try not to drink anything during meals.

2. Take **small bites…chew 25-30 times** per bite (aids digestion again…a lot of digestive enzymes/juices come from chewing). Digestive enzymes are released in the mouth. The intestines don't have to work so hard if we eat more slowly.

3. Drink **hot tea** after meals. Some good teas to aid with digestion are: dandelion, ginger, peppermint, chamomile, green, Senna, and lemon balm

4. Eat a **low acid diet** (avoid acidic things such as citrus fruits, apple cider vinegar, and limit coffee). Eat more alkaline foods.

5. Avoid **"hot foods"** if they bother you. (spicy foods such as hot peppers)

6. Take a **probiotic** to promote the growth of healthy bacteria in your digestive tract. In a probiotic, look for at least 15 billion cultures in a single serving, at least 10 different strains, (some start with the letter L, and some with the letter B). Also, look for delayed release so they will survive the acidity of the stomach and reach your intestines where they are needed. Tip: especially when taking an antibiotic, you NEED to take a probiotic to replace the "good bacteria" that the antibiotic destroyed. This will help to get your immune system healthy so that you don't get sick again. Another tip is to vary the type of probiotic supplement that you purchase from one month to the next so that you will benefit from a variety of strains in your body.

7. **Consume probiotic foods:** Greek yogurt with active or live cultures, kefir, kimchi, blue cheese, aged parmesan cheese, yogurt cheese, acidophilus milk and buttermilk, sauerkraut, tempeh, miso soup, fermented soy sauce.

8. **Prebiotics** are important as well. They nourish the good bacteria: fruits, raw honey, legumes, artichoke, asparagus, oatmeal, brown rice, quinoa, millet, buckwheat, barley, rye, beans and rice are some good prebiotic sources.

9. **Other foods to support your digestive health:** apples, prunes, berries, carrots, Brussels sprouts, broccoli, yams, walnuts, pistachios, salmon, olive oil, sunflower seeds and oil, corn, flax, chickpeas, soy, papaya juice and gooseberry. Also, all antioxidants, anti-inflammatory foods and detoxifying foods are good to include.

10. **Aid digestive disorders and inflammation:** mix together (3 oz. each) aloe Vera juice and pomegranate juice…drink on an empty stomach when you first wake up.

11. Use **peppermint oil** to ease stomach issues. (put drops in tea or 200 mg tablets)

Experiment with Spices to help with digestion:

Relieve Indigestion, bloating and gas: basil, bay leaves, caraway, cardamom, cayenne, fennel, ginger, marjoram, rosemary

Stimulates Digestion: black pepper, chives, cloves, garlic, gentian, horseradish, mustard seed, sage, turmeric

Supplements that might be helpful for digestive issues:

Niacin (B3), krill oil or fish oil, probiotics, red rice yeast extract, coenzyme Q10, garlic, guggul, apple pectin, zinc, and glutamine.

Note: Check with your doctor before adding supplements to your dietary plan. Some medications or health conditions may interact with even healthy supplements.

DAY 7: WEIGHT LOSS WONDERS

Weight loss is a "hot topic" for sure. Today we will learn many tips and tools to make weight loss simple and easy. You will learn how many calories your body uses each day.

Food is the key.

The most powerful tool you have for health and ideal weight is your fork! Learn to look at food as medicine. Eat more whole, real food. The DNA in food "talks" to your cells and provides the building blocks for healthy function.

How many calories do you burn daily?

Take your current weight and multiply by 12. This is how many calories your body uses each day. To lose weight, you must eat less than that amount!

Figure your number out right now and write it down here: _____

Tips for Weight Loss: As you read through this list, highlight the ones that you feel you can make a commitment to incorporate into your new healthy lifestyle:

1. As explained earlier, many people are gluten sensitive. Consider eliminating **wheat** in your diet.

2. **Eliminate** sugar, alcohol, and traditional dairy.

3. Learn to consistently use a **hunger scale.** Think of a scale from 1 to 10 in terms of how hungry you are. An example of a 1 on the scale is how you feel immediately after a huge Thanksgiving meal. A 10 would be how you might feel if you haven't eaten for an entire day. Your goal is to eat when you feel about a 5 or 6 on this scale. When we wait to eat when we are truly very HUNGRY is when we make bad food choices and overeat.

4. Drink a **glass of water** 20 minutes before eating. Don't drink a lot while eating. **Drink warm tea** after eating to aid digestion.

5. Take a 10-minute **power walk** after eating.

6. Keep track of your food and drink intake. This will be discussed further and sample forms will be given. Any method you like is fine, but do it! You are much more likely to make healthful food choices when you keep a food diary.

7. Begin to make the **connection between what you eat and how it makes you feel.** You will begin to notice which foods don't agree with you. Pay attention to headaches, fatigue, or nausea after you eat.

8. Start to think about **WHY you are eating.** Many of us eat out of boredom or habit. We may eat for comfort. Notice your habits and triggers.

9. **Change your mind set.** Begin to eat until you are no longer hungry instead of eating until you feel full. It takes your brain 20 minutes to register to you that you are full. Eat more slowly.

10. **Don't deny yourself things you love.** Try this tip: eat 2 bites of anything you want…follow it with a full glass of water! You'll feel less deprived if you allow yourself this "2 bite treat". This way you can fully enjoy what you love and not feel guilty about it. Savor those bites!

11. Give yourself a **cheat meal** once a week! (not a cheat DAY, a cheat MEAL) The day that you know you are going to have the cheat meal, eat a huge salad once that day. Really eat healthfully and limit your calories the rest of that day so that you can enjoy your cheat meal.

12. Make it a habit to give your body at least a **12 hour "fast"**. So, for example, if you get up at 7 a.m., stop eating at 7 p.m.

13. Another weight loss and fat burning tip is to **exercise first thing in the morning** before eating.

14. Eat foods that keep you **full and satisfied.** Proteins, nuts, seeds, beans, cranberries, tomatoes, eggplant, green leafy vegetables, fiber rich foods.

15. **Coconut oil** aids with weight loss because it increases your metabolism. It is also anti-inflammatory. Try adding it to smoothies.

16. **Morning drink habit:** First thing in the morning, drink a cup of **hot water and lemon.** Follow this with 2 glasses of water. Do this before you allow yourself to drink anything else for the day.

17. Drink **green tea** every day. Keep healthy snacks and tea or water with you!

18. **Eat 5 small meals per day.** The **combination of foods is vital** to keep blood sugar and hormone levels in balance and for weight loss to be able to occur! Always eat all 3 of these together – protein, carbohydrate (non-starchy) and a healthy fat. A sample 3-day meal plan is provided in the Resource section in the back of the book.

19. **Banish artificial sweeteners!** They sabotage weight loss. In fact, they cause weight gain! They trigger the brain to crave sugar, stimulate the bladder, increase insulin and cause hunger cravings.

20. Increase the amount of **greens** that you eat each day. Make half your plate vegetables. You can eat a large volume of vegetables, helping you feel satisfied.

21. Vegetables and Fruits – go for a variety of color daily.

22. **Help to balance your hormones by consuming some of these:** B6, B12, evening primrose oil, cod liver oil and krill oil, broccoli, collard greens, kale, and magnesium.

23. Get into the habit of **weighing yourself** every Friday and Monday. This will help you to stop overeating and binging on the weekends.

More information to support healthy weight loss:

- **Supplements:** Caralluma Fimbriata, Garcinia Cambogia Extract (GCE), EGCG Green Tea Extract, Cacao nibs, guggul, GTF Chromium, grape seed extract, Vitamin C, probiotic, Spanish bee pollen, white bean extract, forskolin, white mulberry. Do your research before deciding to try any new supplement.

- **Teas:** Green, Oolong, Yerba Mate, and Mulberry.

- **Spices & Condiments:** garlic, chili powder, tabasco sauce, salsa, cayenne or ground red pepper, paprika, curry, turmeric, ginger, horseradish, mustard, cinnamon, apple cider vinegar, pesto sauce.

- **Fruits:** Eat a blend of at least 3 fruits first thing in the morning! (one cup total) cherries, pomegranate, golden berry, goji berry, acai berry, grapes, oranges, grapefruit, apples, pears, lemons, limes, blueberries, bananas, cranberries, mango, raspberry, blackberry, pineapple.

- **Vegetables:** Red peppers, sweet potatoes, jalapeno, habaneros, red cayenne chills, broccoli, tomatoes, spinach, asparagus, carrots, kale, all greens, celery.

- **Protein:** almond butter, beans, nuts and seeds, lean beef, tuna, lean turkey, chicken, pork, salmon, tuna, low fat Greek yogurt

- **Other:** Miso soup, sauerkraut, kimchee, fermented soy sauce

- **Drinks:** COLD water, coffee, green tea, red wine, hot water / lemon in the a.m.

- **Whole Grains:** cereals, breads, pasta, oatmeal

- **Healthy Oils/Fats:** extra virgin olive oil, coconut oil, grapeseed oil, canola oil, macadamia nut oil, toasted sesame oil, walnut oil, avocado, olives, dark chocolate, flaxseed, cashews, walnuts, pecans, almonds, pistachios, sunflower seeds, eggs, real organic butter or smart balance butter.

*"Go confidently in the direction of your dreams.
Live the life you have imagined."*

-Henry David Thoreau

CHAPTER 3 RECAP:

You have been creating new healthy habits for 2 weeks now!

This week we learned:

1. **Protein** was discussed on day one of this chapter. You now know how much protein to eat each day and which proteins are lean and healthy.

2. You now know that **fats are important in the diet.** You learned which fats to include in your meal plan.

3. You learned **which carbohydrates are good for you** and that your focus should be to literally make half of your plate veggies. Non-starchy vegetables are the ones that will be the most healthful.

4. **Strengthening and toning** exercises will increase your metabolism and keep your muscles, bones and joints healthy as you age.

5. Having a **gratitude attitude** will enable you to go through your day with a more positive focus. When you look for the good things, you will notice them all around you.

6. You learned many tips and tricks to aid in **digestion** so that you will experience less food related discomfort.

7. **Weight loss suggestions** were discussed on day 7 of this week's lessons. There are many new habits to incorporate in your life that will result in a leaner you.

List some things that you intend to start doing.

_____   _____

_____   _____

_____   _____

_____   _____

_____   _____

List some things that you are going to stop doing.

_____   _____

Identify any roadblocks that you have. What can you do about them? _____

_____

_____

_____

_____

_____

_____

Come up with a plan or solution to your roadblocks. _____

_____

_____

_____

_____

_____

_____

CHAPTER 4 - WEEK 3

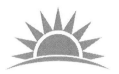

DAY 1:
ULTIMATE HEALTH FOOD DIARY, TIPS & LOGGING

"The only person you are destined to become is the person you decide to be."

-Ralph Waldo Emerson

You have been learning a lot of information about beginning new healthy lifestyle habits and specifics about which foods to include in your meal plans and which to eliminate.

Today, you will be given the Ultimate Health Food Diary and corresponding Tip Sheet. This will make it simple for you to choose meals that will include lean protein, healthy fats and complex carbs.

You will see two styles of logging sheets. These are just examples. Feel free to find your own way of **keeping track of your food and water intake.** There are many apps that you can use on your computer or phone to do this as well.

Use the method that works best for you, but please do keep a food record of some sort. You will have a much greater likelihood of healthful eating if you do!

Make a commitment to eat clean, detoxifying foods.
They cleanse, energize, revive, and nourish your body. You will feel amazing.

Your task is to decide how you are going to keep track of the food and drink that you consume. Begin tomorrow with whatever method you decided on! It's easy! Add this new healthy habit to your daily routine! Check out Sparkpeople.com, Web MD, or Lose it for more ideas and inspiration.

THE ULTIMATE HEALTH FOOD DIARY

You really can eat MORE and lose weight! Follow this guide to get the right combination of foods and nutrition that your body needs. Focus on getting the nutrition IN and don't worry about what to avoid. When you eat more healthfully, you truly will NOT crave so much junk!

SWEET VEGETABLES
(Eat 2 daily – early in the day to reduce cravings for sweets)

Corn   carrots   onions   beets   winter squash   sweet potatoes   yams   pumpkin   parsnips

LEAFY GREEN VEGETABLES - (Unlimited! Eat at least 3 daily)

Broccoli   bok choy   cabbage   kale   collard greens   watercress   mustard greens   dandelion   green cabbage   arugula   endive   chicory   lettuce   mesclun   spinach   swiss chard   beet greens   parsley

ALL OTHER VEGETABLES - (Eat at least 2 daily) *variety of colors

Cauliflower   sea vegetables (nori, wakame, kombu, dulse)   celery   bell peppers   peas   zucchini   tomatoes   radishes   artichoke   asparagus   lima beans   jalapenos   habaneros   red cayenne chilies   eggplant   Brussels sprouts   snow peas   burdock   beets   mushrooms   sauerkraut   fennel   green beans   leeks   potato   avocado   cilantro   cucumber   dandelion   okra   onions   all sprouts

FRUITS - (Eat 3-4 daily) *early in the day   *one cup total

Acai   golden berry   goji berry   blueberries   oranges   bilberry   cranberry   blackberry   prunes   raspberry   strawberry   grapes   plums   cherries   apples   lemons   limes   grapefruit   pears   bananas   tangerines   clementine   kiwi   watermelon   cantaloupe   peaches   strawberry   dates   figs   pomegranate   pineapple   papaya   apricot   guavas   mangoes   nectarines   persimmons   melon

WHOLE GRAINS - (Eat 3-4 daily)

Quinoa   Sorghum   Brown rice   whole grain barley   millet   oats   whole grain corn   whole wheat pasta   rye   whole wheat bread   whole wheat cereal   popcorn   wild rice   buckwheat   bulgur   wheat crackers

PROTEINS - (Eat 3 or 4 oz Servings 3-5 times daily)

Legumes:

adzuki   bean sprouts   fava   garbanzo   kidney   lentils   black   refried

pinto   lima   split pea   tofu, soy

Additional Proteins:

Grass fed beef   organic chicken breast   pork tenderloin   lean steak   fish   tuna

wild salmon   trout   veal turkey   sardines   nuts and seeds   organic eggs

organic Greek yogurt   nut butters   hummus   protein powder

HEALTHY FATS - (Eat 3 -4 daily)

Healthy Oils:

extra virgin olive oil   sesame   sunflower   safflower   peanut   canola   coconut   grapeseed

Additional Fats:

avocado   olives   dark chocolate   flaxseed or flax oil   almond and peanut butter

cashews   walnuts   pecans   almonds   chia seeds   pumpkin seeds   pistachios

sunflower seeds   butter   soy   ghee   granola

ORGANIC DAIRY/DAIRY ALTERNATIVE - (2-4 Servings daily)

Greek yogurt   hard cheeses (Mozzarella, Cheddar, Parmesan, Colby)   Organic Milk

Kefir   low fat sour cream or cottage cheese

Any Almond, Coconut, Rice, Cashew or Hemp Milk Products

WATER - (6-8 Glasses daily)

X   X   X   X   X   X   X   X

OTHER BEVERAGES SHOULD BE TEA OR COFFEE

ULTIMATE HEALTH TIPS AND RECOMMENDATIONS:

1. **Keep a record** of what you eat and drink – you are much more likely to stick to a healthy food plan when you do. What you are eating too little of or too much of will be easily recognized by keeping a visual record. **Tip:** use the Ultimate Health Food LOG on the previous page for several days in a row by using different colors of ink to represent different days of the week.

2. Drink hot water and lemon first thing in the morning. **The first thing you should eat after that is protein and fruits.** This is natures way of detoxing your body. This is your break "fast". Try to stop eating 3 hours before bedtime and let your body be without food for 12 hours (fasting).

3. Use a **hunger scale** of 1-10. To avoid over eating, try to eat when you feel like you are about at a 4, 5, or 6 on the scale. This will also keep your metabolism going. Additionally, begin to pay attention to your emotions when you eat. When do you eat? Why are you eating? Bored, sad, celebrating, stressed, mindless snacking?

4. Strive to **eat 4-6 small meals** throughout the day (eat every 3 or 4 hours). The combination of nutrients in each meal is important. **Always combine** a healthy protein, non-starcy carbohydrate and a healthy fat together! Remember to include a variety of colorful vegetables and fruits, whole grains, and a variety of healthy fats.

5. **Make ½ of your plate vegetables** at every meal. Organic if possible, then in this order…FRESH, frozen, canned. Consume some raw and some cooked daily.

6. Drink **water** all through the day. Being hydrated keeps your from haivng cravings. Carry water with you ALWAYS. Add lime, lemon, or berries to the water for variety. Drink 2 glasses of water every morning and one before all meals.

7. **Move..move..move!** Get some exercise. 30 to 60 minutes 5 days of the week is optimal.

8. **Superstar Supplements:** take a good **whole food** multivitamin and other supplements based on your diet and health issues. Most people would benefit from a multivitamin, probiotic, D-3, Fish Oil and B Complex. Consult your physician before taking anything new.

9. Eliminate Artificial Sweeteners! try these **natural sweeteners:** stevia, xylitol, rice syrup, raw organic honey, 100% maple syrup.

More: water, teas (especially green), whole grains, leafy greens, variety of colorful vegetables and fruits. A variety of lean protein sources, home cooked meals, organic, exercise, healthy relationships, gratitude, and joy.

Less: red meat, alcohol, tobacco products, sugar, coffee, dairy, and caffeine.

Eliminate: white products (pasta, bread, potatoes), fast food, soda, "diet" products of any kind, processed foods, refined foods, pre-packaged and boxed foods, chemicals, preservatives, transfats, artifical sweeteners of any kind, pesticides, hormones and antibiotics in foods (meats, poultry, vegetables, fruits, and dairy), empty calories, and unhealthy habits.

Food Diary - Option 2

On the right of this form, record your "mood" for feelings from the foods you eat and beverages you drink. Doing this will enable to you to realize how different foods affect you. Do you have more or less energy? How is your digestion after eating certain types of foods? How is your sleep affected? Examples of adjectives to use: tired, energized, anxious, uncomfortable, jittery, alert, satiated, calm, nauseated. Also, rate your hunger from 1 -10, with a 10 being "extremely hungry!"

                          Mood/Effects Noticed   **Hunger Scale: 1-10**

Breakfast: _____   _____
(fruit, protein)

Snack: _____   _____
(protein, healthy fat, complex carbohydrate)

Lunch: _____   _____
(omega 3, lean protein, healthy fat, complex carbohydrate (incorporate Vitamin C also)

Snack: _____   _____
(small serving –again healthy fat, lean protein, complex carbohydrate)

Dinner: _____   _____
(protein, complex carbohydrate, healthy fat – add zinc in the meal)

Snack: _____   _____
(try not to eat 3 hours before bedtime (if you do, have a complex carbohydrate)

Circle the X's below as you consume them each day

Water (6 daily)   x x x x x x   *drink a glass of water before eating anything!

MUFA (4 daily)   x x x x   *drink warm tea after meals!

Grains (4 daily)   x x x x   *grains can be completely eliminated!

Vegetables (5 daily)   x x x x x   *variety of color with fruits / veggies!

Fruits (4 daily)   x   x   x   x   *eat these the first part of the day

Proteins (3-5 daily)   x   x   x   x   *eat small amounts of protein often (3-4 oz)

Dairy (2 daily)   x   x   *use dairy alternatives

Healthy fats (MUFA): oils, olives, nuts/seeds, avocado, dark chocolate, peanut butter or nut butter, flaxseed, cashews, walnuts, pecans, almonds, pistachios, sunflower seeds, semi-sweet chocolate chips

Proteins: lean meats, nut butters, fish, eggs, milk, leafy greens, whole grains, beans, nuts & seeds, lentils

Grains: quinoa, sorghum, oats, barley, brown rice, whole wheat breads and pasta, beans, peas, nuts/seeds

Zinc: seafood, organic meats, spinach, pumpkin seeds, cashews, cocoa, chocolate, mushrooms, beans

Vitamin C: chili peppers bell peppers, guavas, dark leafy greens, broccoli, cauliflower, Brussels sprouts, kiwi, papaya, oranges, strawberries.

DAY 2: GRAINS

Grains are the topic of the day today. As I mentioned before, a very small percent of the population has celiac disease and are 100% gluten intolerant. However, a large percentage of us are gluten sensitive.

Symptoms of gluten sensitivity are brain fog, inability to focus and concentrate, belly bloat and an uncomfortable feeling in your stomach, headaches, nausea and lack of energy. If you suspect you might be gluten sensitive, go for 2 weeks without gluten and see how you feel. If you do feel better, you will know that it is best for you to eliminate grains from your diet completely.

The benefits of grains:

1. Good source of nutrition (iron, fiber, vitamins E and B, and enzymes).
2. Grains help keep you full and satisfied because your body absorbs them slowly.
3. They are a good energy source for the body.

Below are some grains that do NOT contain gluten. Use these most often.

1. Brown or Wild Rice
2. Buckwheat
3. Amaranth
4. Cornmeal
5. Millet
6. Quinoa
7. Sorghum
8. Arrowroot, Teff, Montina
9. Rolled Oats and Whole Oats (but in most manufacturing, they could be contaminated with gluten due to contact with other products).
10. Gluten Free: pasta, cereal, pretzels, chips, soy, potato, beans, flax and nut flours.

These grains DO contain gluten:

1. Barley
2. Bulgur (cracked wheat)
3. Couscous

4. Kamut

5. Rye Berries or Wheat Berries

6. Spelt

Tip from my Kitchen: I use quinoa in recipes instead of "meat". Quinoa is the oldest grain in the world. It is very healthy and very versatile. My favorites are the flavored blends such as parmesan or garlic. You can purchase quinoa that you cook (be sure to rinse it first), or you can get it in pouches that are ready to eat. You can add quinoa or quinoa and rice blends in stir fry, soups, or you can eat it as a side dish or even a cereal. It will help keep you full and satisfied! Give it a try!

Below are my favorite recipes using quinoa or oats.

I consistently make either stir fry vegetables or vegetable soup every week. Sometimes I add lean beef, turkey burger or even tofu! Other times I add a blend of quinoa and brown rice. There is such a variety of colorful vegetables in every serving. What a delicious health boost! Make this a new habit for yourself as well.

Want to try to start incorporating tofu in your meals? This is a great way to do it! Make tofu more like the consistency of hamburger by putting oil in a pan and browning and crumbling the tofu just like you would hamburger. Try it in the recipes for soup or stir fry! P.S. You don't have to tell your family and friends that tofu was an ingredient!

No Bake Energy Treats

These are simple to make! Mix these ingredients, roll into balls & refrigerate.

- 1 cup dry oatmeal (old fashioned rolled oats)
- 1/2 cup semi-sweet MINI chocolate chips
- 1/2 cup peanut butter or almond butter
- 1/4 cup ground flaxseed or any seed mix (optional)
- 1/3 cup organic honey
- 1 teaspoon vanilla

Make them your own! Add anything you want to: coconut, raisins, dates, cranberries

To make them roll up easier: Stir the ingredients and put in refrigerator for about 20 minutes, then roll into balls. Put coconut oil on your hands so you can roll them up more easily.

Immune Boosting Soup:

Base: you can use either tomato juice, V-8, organic chicken broth or vegetable broth

Combine:
Bell peppers (yellow, red and orange), l/2 cup lemon juice, 1 cup sliced carrots, ½ tsp. minced garlic, ½ tsp. minced ginger, ½ bunch of red onion, l/2 pound shitake mushrooms, chicken stock, 2 tbsp. brewed soy sauce, 1 block of tofu, red, black or white beans, cooked quinoa, and black pepper/salt to taste.

Optional: jalapeno peppers (if you can take the heat!)

Slimming Soup

No need to measure anything! You can use a crock pot for this, or make on the stovetop. Use tomato juice as the base. Cut up cabbage, red cabbage and onion. Add in as many fresh or frozen vegetables as you like. (green beans, peas, corn, peppers, mushrooms, etc.). Add a dash of Worchester sauce. Add garlic, beans, anything you like and salt/pepper to taste). This is a wonderful way to get a variety of veggies in your daily diet. Add quinoa to this to make it more filling and energy boosting.

Quinoa and Stir Fry Veggies:

Prepare the quinoa as directed and set aside. I first sauté onions, peppers and garlic. Next, I add a large bag of frozen stir fry vegetables. Add any spices that you like. When completed, stir in the quinoa. I make a huge pan each week. This is a wonderful, easy way to get healthy grains and a variety of colorful vegetables in one simple meal.

How do you feel about grains? Do you suspect you are gluten sensitive? If so, start tomorrow with the 2 week "no gluten test" and see. It will be evident to you at the end of 2 weeks if you feel better or not.

DAY 3:
IMMUNE BOOSTING WITH SUPERFOODS AND ANTIOXIDANTS

"Let food be thy medicine and medicine by thy food"

- Hippocrates

Your immune system functions as your body's fighter jets. Ideally, you will give your body real, whole, nutrient dense food to build a strong defense system.

Mother Nature gave us antioxidants and superfoods as the fuel to use to fight free radicals and disease. Superfoods and antioxidants are nutrient dense and packed full of health enhancing properties. They fight infection, enhance the immune system and protect against diseases such as osteoporosis, heart disease, cancer, diabetes, and respiratory infections.

The reason we need to focus on making vegetables (plants) half of our plate whenever we eat anything is because they contain powerful **phytonutrients.**

There are 3 types of phytonutrients:

1. **Flavonoids** cause antioxidant activity. They have the ability to modify the body's reaction to allergens, viruses and carcinogens. Examples are fruits, vegetables, tea, red wine, and grape juice.

2. **Carotenoids** are the pigments in fruits and vegetables. Focus on getting in all of the colors you can every day. Red, Orange, Yellow, Green, Purple, Blue…they all have different health properties.

3. **Polyphenols** are compounds found in a variety of plants that aid in development of your body's immune system. The best sources are onion, apple, tea, red wine, red grapes, grape juice, strawberries, raspberries, blueberries, cranberries and nuts.

Remember, you literally are what you eat. Begin to look at food differently.

Change your thinking - Begin to eat to live rather than live to eat!

The Best Super Foods:
The Very Highest Antioxidant Rich Sources

1. Goji Berries (Wolfberry)
2. White Mulberry
3. Gooseberry and Golden Berry
4. Acai (AH sigh EE)
5. Blueberries
6. Sweet potatoes
7. Broccoli
8. Cacao (raw dark chocolate) add the nibs or powder to smoothies!
9. Camu berry
10. Spirulina, Chlorella, and all AFA blue-green algae
11. Sea vegetables (kelp, dulse, nori, hijuki,)
12. Bee products (try to buy local honey close to your location)
13. Medicinal mushrooms (reishi, king oyster and shiitake) *check out powdered blends of many varieties of mushrooms
14. Tomatoes (especially when combined with oil) *Salsa is an ideal snack!

Other Antioxidant Super Foods:

- **Drinks:** concord grape juice, red wine, white tea, green tea, apple cider vinegar, aloe juice, cod liver oil, omega 3 oils, hemp oil, pomegranate juice, dark cherry juice, acai juice, Superfood juice blends. (look for 100% juice, no sugar added)

- **Nuts, Seeds, Grains:** walnuts, almonds, brazil nuts, pumpkin seeds, flax seeds, chia seeds, hemp seeds, sesame seeds, sunflower, quinoa, oatmeal

- **Fruits:** bilberry, cranberry, blackberry, black currants, pomegranate, prunes, raspberry, strawberry, grapes, plums, cherries, apples, lemons, limes, kiwi fruit, apricots, coconut, avocado, and elderberry.

- **Beans:** red kidney beans, pinto beans, black beans, soy beans, black bean refried

- **Dairy/ Dairy Alternatives:** Greek yogurt, organic eggs, Almond Milk, Hemp Milk, Rice Milk, Coconut Milk, Cashew Milk, Soy Milk, organic milk.

- **Vegetables:** Carrots, artichoke, celery, kale, spinach, broccoli, parsley, Swiss Chard, bell peppers, zucchini, tomatoes, asparagus, Brussels sprouts, cauliflower, beets, mushrooms, green beans, sweet potato, cucumber, Bok choy.

Be sure to eat cruciferous foods too (broccoli, cauliflower, kale, collards, Brussels sprouts, cabbage, and baby arugula)

When you sit down to **plan meals,** make sure you **include the super foods and antioxidant foods** that you have read about today. Get a variety of colors in every day of both fruits and vegetables. Build a super strong immune system to be able to fight off illness.

Remember: *REAL food expires in a week.* If something could sit on a shelf for 5 years and you could still eat it…do you want to? LIVING food will nourish your body and give it the building blocks that it needs.

Want to FEEL healthy, vital, full of energy and alive?
EAT REAL FOOD.

Raw Food Diet:

Following a raw food diet is a very strict way of eating. On this plan, you only eat raw food in its natural form: berries, vegetables, roots, flowers, sea vegetables, nuts, seeds, sprouts and water. Eating real, whole, nutritious food has many benefits. You are eliminating poisons and toxins of chemicalized and processed products. A raw food diet is advised for all kinds of health issues such as cancer, diabetes, cholesterol, high blood pressure, and obesity. If you want to, give this a try for 2 to 4 weeks. See how you feel! Attempt to eat purely organic during this time.

DAY 4: FITNESS TIPS FOR MAXIMUM CALORIE BURN

Let's learn more about the best ways to exercise.

The best tip I can give you is to vary the type of workouts and exercises that you do. Your body will get different benefits from a variety of things. Don't get stuck in a rut.

Fitness Tips to maximize weight loss and fat burning:

1. If you can **exercise first thing in the morning,** before eating, you will maximize the calorie burn. Your body will be in the fat burning state after not eating for about 12 hours. So, if you don't eat anything at least 2 hours before bed and you get up first thing in the morning and exercise this will be very beneficial for weight loss! Drink your lemon water and a glass of water before you exercise and another glass of water immediately after exercise. What a start to your day!

2. Remember to add **strength training** to your weekly routine. By toning up, you are increasing your metabolism 24 hours a day.

3. Take a **10-minute power walk** after eating whenever possible.

4. Instead of exercising at a steady speed, vary your pace.

    To illustrate why varying your pace makes sense and is better for a more effective workout think of it like this: When you drive your car on the interstate with the cruise set at 70 miles per hour, the car burns fuel. But by going at that same steady pace, it is energy efficient. When you make the car go faster and slower constantly, it uses more fuel! Your body is the same way. Burn more calories and get more fat burning by varying your pace when you work out!

5. **Blast More Fat with Interval Training!** You can take an organized class utilizing these methods or simply make up your own workout. Interval Training is a way of exercising where you alternate fast paced activity for 30 or 40 seconds, followed by a slower pace to bring the heart rate back down. Examples of interval training follow.

Sample 35 Minute Walk/Jog Interval Training Workout:

10 Minutes	Walk at a brisk pace to warm up
8 Minutes	Perform 8 One Minute Intervals
	30 -seconds medium pace, 30- seconds fast
	(the fast segment should be as fast as you can go)
	REPEAT this 7 more times
5 Minutes	Walk at your normal pace and get your heartrate down
7 Minutes	Do Some Strength Exercises (Bicep, Triceps, Shoulders, Back, Abs, Core)
5 Minute	Light stretches for flexibility

You can also do this type of Interval workout with **movements** such as jumping jacks, push- ups, burpees, mountain climbers, lunges, etc. See below!

Examples of an interval workout using exercises:

5-minute Warm up		*March in place, knee lifts, just move until you begin to sweat!
Movement 1	Jumping Jacks	40 seconds full out, 20-second rest
Movement 2	Jump Rope	40 seconds full out, 20-second rest
Movement 3	Left Leg Lunges	40 seconds full out, 20-second rest
Movement 4	Burpees	40 seconds full out, 20-second rest
Movement 5	Right leg Lunges	40 seconds full out, 20-second rest
Movement 6	Mountain Climbers	40 seconds full out, 20-second rest
Movement 7	Squats	40 seconds full out, 20-second rest
Movement 8	Plank Hold	40 seconds full out, 20-second rest

One Minute Drink / Rest Break and Repeat this one more time

Cool down/ Stretch/ Drink Water

On different days, vary your workout. A 5-day weekly sample is below:

Day	Type of Activity	Fast	Slower
Monday	Walk/Jog Interval Training	30 Sec.	30 Sec.
Tuesday	Interval Workout Using Exercises	45 Sec.	15 Sec.
Thursday	Stationary Bike Workout	60 Sec.	30 Sec.
Friday	Interval Workout Using Exercises	50 Sec.	10 Sec.
Sunday	Treadmill Workout	40 Sec.	20 Sec.

Benefits of Interval Training (vary fast/slow pace):

1. It increases your **metabolism**
2. It increases **fat burning**
3. It **increases calorie burning** even after the workout
4. You get a quality workout with a **shorter amount of time** invested!

There is no right or wrong.

It doesn't matter HOW you move, just THAT you MOVE!

1. Use any **exercise machine** that you like.
2. Just **walk!**
3. Take a **class** (Zumba, water aerobics, cycling, kickboxing, swim, whatever you like!)
4. Hire a **personal trainer** to get you off to a great start
5. Find a **program** to join for **support.**
6. Do a **variety** of movements each week. **Vary the pace and type** of activity!
7. **MOVE!** Just Move!
8. More bang for your investment of time. Look for ways to maximize the workout. **Multi-task!** For example, instead of standing still and doing bicep curls, you could do alternating lunges backward as you do the curls. Look for ways to use more than one muscle group at the same time.
9. On the interval workouts, during the "fast" cycle, work HARD!
10. **If it doesn't challenge you, it can't change you! Short bursts of intensity will result in maximum results.**

DAY 5:
JOURNALING BASICS
MORNING AND EVENING

Journaling is a powerful tool. Allowing time for personal reflection is helpful.
It is a type of therapy.
I hope that I'll inspire you to give it a try.

Journaling - Morning

If you make time earlier in the day to allow yourself to deal with your stressors, concerns, and worries, you will train yourself to be more relaxed in the evening. Another benefit of allowing yourself to have some quiet and solitude each day to calmly think and focus on the issues in your life is that it will allow clarity and insight. Answers and solutions will come to you when you give your troubles and issues more intentional thought.

Many of us have trouble falling asleep at night because we can't quiet our mind. We can go through our day and not dwell on the issues and problems in our lives because we are busy and our minds are occupied. But, when we wind down at the end of the day to try to sleep, we just can't stop the negativity and worry from entering our minds.

Solution: Early in the day, find an opportunity to sit down in a quiet place. Allow 10-15 minutes to yourself. Use the following to focus, think, and write about what is on your mind and in your heart. Jot down whatever comes to your mind. No one will see this but you.

My concerns are:_____

_____

I am worried about:_____

_____

I am upset or fearful about: _____

_____

These things need my time and attention: _____

_____

My "to do" list for today is: _____

_____

I need to pray about: _____

_____

I need a solution to: _____

_____

Now…go back over what you've written about. Cross through the ones you cannot do anything about. Pray about those and let them go. Now look at the ones you can do something about. Decide on an action plan to deal with them.

This works for me! At night, when those upsetting thoughts enter my mind, I literally visualize taking a large eraser and wiping it across my forehead. I remind myself that I dealt with those things earlier and I refuse to let the negative things consume me. With repetition and practice, this will begin to work more effectively.

To recap: EARLY in the day, write down your worries and concerns. After you have written them all down, go back and mark out the ones you cannot control, fix or change. Then, for the things you can "fix", try to come up with an action plan.

Train your brain to focus on these things early in the day…and wipe them away late at night. The more you practice this, the more effective it will become.

Writing is a form of release and healing. Give it a try.

> *"We are what we repeatedly do.*
> *You will never change your life until you change something you do daily.*
> *The secret of your success is found in your daily routine."*
>
> —John C. Maxwell

> *"You are perfect. You are complete.*
> *Your inner voice always knows what to do, but it is a quiet voice.*
> *You can only hear the whisperings of your inner voice—your inner compass—when you turn down the volume of your fears, your regrets, your resentments and the fear-based advice your neighbors are so willing to give you."*
>
> —Jonathan Lockwood Huie

Evening Journaling Ritual

Keep a journal by your bed. Make this a part of your bedtime ritual. Consider doing this with your loved ones as well. End the day thinking of positive things. What a perfect way to end the day and go to sleep thinking of the good happenings of the day.

Victory: (something you are proud of) _____

_____

_____

_____

Laughter: (something amusing that happened today) _____

_____

_____

_____

_____

Gratitude: (something you are thankful for today) _____

_____

_____

_____

_____

Kindness: (what have you done for someone else today?)_____

_____

_____

_____

_____

Relaxation: (something relaxing you did for yourself today)_____

_____

_____

_____

_____

Spirituality: What did you do today to nourish your soul or uplift your spirit?

Examples: meditation, inspirational reading, devotion, bible reading, imagery, relaxing music, time in nature

_____

_____

_____

_____

Happiness: Be sure to do something every day that makes you happy. What did you do today? _____

_____

_____

_____

_____

DAY 6: HOME COOKING

You will be amazed at how easy it is and how much better you feel!

Home cooking is the most wonderful thing you can do for the health of yourself and your family! It doesn't take that much time. The only way to know the quality of the food you consume is to buy and prepare it yourself. Even if you order a "healthy food" at a restaurant, you have no idea of the quality of the food or the oils used in preparation. Make the commitment to cook more at home. It's better than take-out!

We all live very busy lives. We tend to eat very unhealthy because we need to grab what is fast, cheap, convenient, and easy. This is seldom nutritious! Home cooking does not have to be time consuming. Make the decision to do it!

Planning Meals and Snacks

Set aside 20-30 minutes a week to plan meals and snacks for the entire week. Make your grocery list based on your meal and snack plan. As mentioned before, you should plan two weeks of meals and snacks with corresponding grocery lists. Then simply repeat! There is magic in this simplicity, routine and repetition. When you take the guesswork out of what you are going to eat, you make better choices! It's that simple.

Grocery Shopping

Using the list that you've already made, do your grocery shopping once a week. Don't go to the grocery store when you are hungry. Drink a glass of water and eat a healthy snack before you go. Chew gum while you're at the store. You're less likely to grab unhealthy things at the checkout aisle if you are chewing gum. It also reduces hunger and thirst.

Shop the perimeters of the store first. You've probably noticed that the healthiest foods are around the outside perimeter. For quality and freshness, choose in this order when making food choices: fresh, frozen, canned.

Become a Label Reading Expert!

At every store trip, choose one or two foods to really read the labels to be sure you are choosing a healthy option. Look at fat, calories from fat, servings per container, watch for hidden sugars and pay attention to the salt content.

Try to buy local whenever possible.

Take advantage of farmer's markets and local farms for as much of your food as possible. Buy in season and local. Did you know that many foods at our grocery stores were picked before they were ripe? Many foods travel 1500 miles or more to get to our local stores.

Buy Organic as much as you can.

Each week at the grocery store, I check to see what is organic and on sale! Choose those for sure! The rule of thumb is if a fruit or vegetable can be peeled, you usually don't need to buy organic. **I notice a tremendous difference in the taste of organic apples, carrots, peppers, blueberries and strawberries!** They won't look as "perfect", but oh my, the taste!

Now, let's talk about some time saver tips for home cooking!

1. Set aside two 1 1/2 hour **blocks of time for cooking**. The meal preparation and healthy snack preparation can be done in about 3 hours a week! This will be time well spent. I find this hard to believe, but I truly prefer to eat my own healthy food than food I eat at a restaurant. I feel better when I eat my own cooking. I never thought I'd say that, but it's true.

2. Every time you cook, prepare **2 protein sources and 4 vegetables.** This way you have those foods to mix and match meals for several days. You can also prepare a healthy grain if you want to such as wild rice or quinoa.

3. While your foods are baking or cooking, use the wait time to do your **snack preparation**. Clean and cut veggies and put in baggies. Clean fruits and put those in baggies as well. Make some baggies with a variety of nuts and seeds. Since a serving size is so small with nuts/seeds, I add popcorn for volume.

   *You will be much more likely to eat healthfully and snack wisely if you have these healthy options clean, prepared and ready to grab!

4. **Enlist friends and family** to help you with this! Make it fun.

5. **The freezer is your friend!** Another time saver and money saver is to stock up on foods when you find them on sale. Make more than you need for the week and freeze the extra to use later.

DAY 7:
BREAKFAST MAGIC

Simple   Easy   Nutritious   Delicious

The Magic Healthful Breakfast is simple and easy. Every day for breakfast, have a variety of fruits and a protein. That's it!

My two favorite ways to do this is to have a smoothie or overnight oatmeal.

Smoothie Directions

There are many recipes that you can go by to make healthy smoothies. I don't usually use a recipe, I simply use the guide below. There is no right or wrong, just change it up every day! Smoothies are easy to make. Be cautious of the sugar content however! Some smoothies are very high calorie. Eliminate added sugar.

Choose a Base: Add one or more of these: Greek yogurt, coconut milk, almond milk, rice milk, hemp milk, goat's milk, soy milk, cashew milk, tofu, cooked white beans, avocado.

Liquid Mixer: Water, coconut water, ice, vegetable juice, carrot juice, grapefruit juice, orange juice, apple juice, pomegranate juice, cranberry juice, or any low sugar fruit juice blend.

Fruits: Your goal is to get about **1 cup of fruit** in…first thing in the morning (in this one cup, have a variety of at least **3 different fruits**) Fresh fruit or frozen fruit is fine. Try to find a frozen blend with 3 or more different fruits! Blueberries, blackberries, raspberries, strawberries, banana, mango, papaya, lime, oranges, lemon, pineapple, cherries… any fruits you like are fine.

Veggies: Sliced cabbage, Kale, spinach, broccoli, any greens are good to add in your smoothie. Another great boost is a super greens powdered blend.   *freezing the greens will mellow the flavor of them if you are trying to incorporate them into your smoothies.

Sweetener: To add sweetness, try orange zest, cinnamon, almond extract, unsweetened cocoa, pumpkin puree, or coconut oil. Other options (but they are higher in calorie) are honey, 100% fruit juice, agave nectar or 100% maple syrup.

Health Boosts you might add:

Greens: Powdered super greens will provide a wonderful nutrition boost. They have the sea algae, wheat grasses, and many trace elements and vitamins.

Protein: A whey or pea protein powder is a great health boost to add. Other options are almond butter, peanut butter or any other nut butter.

Seeds: Add ground seeds: chia, pumpkin flax, sunflower, flax, sesame, hemp

Oils: Cod liver oil, Omega 3 swirl, krill oil, coconut oil, flax oil

Overnight Oats

Just like with smoothies, you can find many recipes for overnight oats. There is no real need for a recipe though. See below for directions!

In container (I use a small round bowl or a mason jar), layer these ingredients:

1. Old fashioned 100% whole wheat rolled **oats**

2. Put on top of the oats some **cinnamon** if you want to

3. On top of that, add any healthy "milk" that you like such as almond milk, rice milk, cashew milk, coconut milk, soy milk, goat's milk.

    *add just enough milk to moisten the oats.

4. On top of that, add the 3 different **fruits**

5. Add a **sweetener** or a **health boost i**f you want (same ones as listed for the smoothies)   *I usually add a powdered 6 seed blend and honey

6. Top with Greek **yogurt** or any yogurt (vanilla works best I think)

7. Put in the refrigerator…**no cooking needed!** The next day, stir and **enjoy!**

Reminder: Your goal is to make breakfast be 3 fruits (1 cup total) and a protein.

You are not limited to traditional breakfast foods. Other options might be:

- 100% whole wheat cereal and fruit
- Cooked oatmeal and fruit
- Peanut butter sandwich, ½ banana, ½ apple, ½ orange
- Trail mix, and cheese
- Almond butter, ½ banana, ½ apple, cranberries
- Egg, cheese, and mixed fruit
- Whole wheat bagel and mixed fruit
- Low fat yogurt with mixed fruit and granola
- Hummus on wheat pita bread and mixed fruit

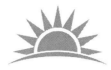

CHAPTER 4 RECAP:

This week you have learned so many new healthy habits. Week by week you are gaining so much information and developing new lifestyle changes. Keep it up!

As a reminder, let's review this week's new tips:

1. **Food Combinations Matter.** Always combine a lean protein, a healthy fat and a complex carbohydrate when you eat.

2. You learned **which grains are the healthiest.** If it is white, don't bite! Eliminate white bread, pasta, potatoes, etc.

3. Your **immune system** is your defense system against disease. By including nutrient dense **superfoods and antioxidants,** you create strong healthy cells, tissues and organs.

4. You learned **ways of exercising** to maximize calorie burning, fat burning and to minimize the time required to get a good workout. The key is to constantly change the pace when you exercise.

5. New **journaling** habits were explained. Some entries are best to do early in the day and some late at night.

6. **Home cooking** is a must. Lots of time savers and tips were given.

7. There is **magic in breakfast!** It should be a protein and a variety of fruits. Many options are available and many health boosts were explained.

List some things that you intend to start doing.

_____   _____
_____   _____
_____   _____
_____   _____
_____   _____

List some things that you are going to stop doing.

_____   _____

_____   _____

_____   _____

_____   _____

_____   _____

Identify any roadblocks that you have. What can you do about them? Come up with a plan or solution to your roadblocks.

_____

_____

_____

_____

_____

_____

_____

CHAPTER 5 - WEEK 4

DAY 1: DISEASE PREVENTION

In *Healthy Living by Design*, you are learning about so many things that make you **happy, healthy, and well.** By now, you are getting the idea that **moderation and balance in all things** is what we all want to achieve.

Probably the single most important thing you can do to help with prevention of disease is to **nourish your body with healthy foods and pure water.** Imbalances in the body lead to disease. **Heart disease and cancer** are at the top of the list in causes of death. You can greatly reduce your chances of being affected by heart disease, cancer and other illnesses by making good lifestyle choices.

> *"Put your future in good hands- your own."*
> - Author Unknown

Disease is caused by many factors: (many of these ARE in your control)

- Not living in a healthy physical environment
- Genetic make-up
- Lack of proper nutrition (balance of protein, fats, carbohydrates, purified water)
- Toxins (chemicals, toxins, cleaners, pollutants)
- Lack of stress management techniques
- Lack of quality sleep, rest and relaxation
- Use of tobacco; excess alcohol or drug use
- Lack of meaning and purpose to your life (meaningful career and hobbies)

- Deficiency in play, bliss, joy (positive people live on average 7 years longer!)
- Not having healthy relationships or a sense of belonging, caring, nurturing

The **digestive system is at the core of your health.** Most of your immune system is in your "gut". It is important to take a probiotic supplement. Eat foods that support the digestive system (fiber, water, and fermented foods).

Remember that your health and well-being are all encompassing. The **mind, body, and spirit are all connected.** Integrative, holistic health is key - what affects one, affects all.

Hidden inflammation in the body is the root cause of much disease!

The underlying cause of chronic illness is inflammation. The Ancient Greeks referred to this inflammation as an internal fire. This inflammation can linger for many years and will attack the body. It can attack the brain, heart, or other organs. Inflammation is a key factor in cancer, heart disease, Alzheimer's, obesity, type 2 diabetes, asthma, allergies, and all other diseases ending with the suffix "itis".

The macronutrients you consume (the carbohydrates, proteins and fats) can increase or decrease the inflammation in your body. These foods in turn create hormonal responses in the body. These hormones are insulin, glucagon, and eicosanoids. Insulin is a storage hormone stimulated by the carbohydrates in a meal. Overeating carbohydrates then makes us fat and keeps us fat.

*Remember that **food can be medicine.***

Food changes everything! Have you ever noticed that **most Americans are overweight, but malnourished?** This is because most people eat modern day convenience "foods" that do not contain vitamins and minerals. So, our bodies CRAVE something else to eat, so we eat and eat and eat…but still we crave more because our bodies are not getting what they need to renew and regenerate and perform bodily functions.

Example: If you are eating nutritious calories, you are noticing that you don't crave as much "junk". Magically, you are satisfied with less because your body is getting what it needs.

What you eat and drink determines the quality of your cells, tissues, and organs. Ideally, half of our diet would come from raw, whole foods (foods that would expire in a week).

Foods that cause inflammation! Stay away from these:

- Meats that are **grilled or fried** at **high temperature** (blackened foods are not healthy…they are carcinogenic)
- **Omega-6 fatty acids:** corn, sunflower, safflower, soybean and cottonseed oils, many fried foods, many processed snack foods, margarine, more than 4 or 5 egg yolks a week.
- Food that come in a **box, processed** lunch meats
- **Non-organic** meats, fruits, vegetables and dairy products.
- **Limit Grains**
- **Avoid "white"** products (sugar, bread, potatoes, pastas). These foods have little or no nutritional value and are empty calories, robbing your body of the building blocks it needs to heal and nourish itself.

Inflammation Fighters!

- Consume **Omega 3 foods and fermented foods:** cod liver oil, flax oil, extra virgin olive oil, canola oil, sardines, herring, wild salmon, tuna, trout, avocado, nuts and seeds, kefir, kimchee, miso, tempeh, pickles, sauerkraut, and olives.
- Eat a **variety of colors of all the antioxidant and super foods** we have talked about earlier. Some reminders are tri-color peppers, onion, garlic, mushrooms, beans, tomatoes, broccoli, cherries, blueberries, peaches, oranges, pears, apples, grapes, nuts, asparagus, cabbage, kale, romaine, spinach, carrots, cranberries, cocoa.
- **Powdered Super Greens** that contain seaweed and grasses: you can put them in smoothies, stir fry, soups) chlorophyll, chlorella, spirulina, wild blue green algae, barley grass, wheat grass, rye grass
- Incorporate these **anti-inflammatory agents** into your daily life: evening primrose oil, coconut oil, ginger, rosemary, curcumin, vitamin c, garlic, turmeric, cloves, parsley, cilantro, cardamom, basil, cinnamon, probiotic supplement, aloe Vera juice mixed with pomegranate juice, baby aspirin if you are over 40.
- **Other lifestyle helpers to fight inflammation:** far infrared sauna, massage, acupuncture, low impact exercise (water aerobics, yoga, Pilates, walking).

Food changes everything…. literally. What you eat and drink determines the quality of your cells, tissues, and organs. Ideally, half of your diet would come from raw, whole foods (foods that would expire in a week).

We all should consume foods high in **fiber** and **omega-3 essential fatty acids**. They boost the function of your immune system. These are whole foods which are a factory of minerals, vitamins, phytochemicals, and nutrients. Omega 3 rich foods boost brain function, fight inflammation, cancer, and heart disease. Refined foods are foods that are full of chemicals and is processed and altered (example...a meal that comes in a box, foods with added hormones, antibiotics, pesticides, fertilizers, is genetically altered in some way).

Reminder – Some Examples of Healthy Whole Foods

Vegetables:	Carrots, broccoli, lettuces, sweet potatoes, cauliflower, spinach, peppers, kale
Fruits:	Bananas, apples, strawberries, blueberries, grapes, watermelon, peaches
Grains:	Quinoa, brown rice, oatmeal, barley, buckwheat, millet, sprouted grains
Greens:	Broccoli, collards, kale, spinach, chard, cabbage, dark lettuce, micro-algae, and grasses found in powdered super greens
Broth:	Organic vegetable, chicken and bone broth
Legumes:	Fermented soy, all beans, peas and lentils
Dairy:	Organic Dairy is fine, but diary alternatives are better for you: Almond, Soy, Cashew, Hemp, Coconut Milk and products
Fish/Meat	Organic, crass fed, cage free. Try to buy from local farms when possible.
Other:	Nuts and seeds, spices such as turmeric and ginger, garlic, onion, chives

An Alkaline Diet is Beneficial for Disease Prevention

With most disease, an **alkaline diet** is necessary to purify and detoxify the body. Disease thrives in an acidic environment. So, we can help control the acidity of our blood by consuming a lot of alkaline foods and limiting the acidic ones. Once digested and broken down by the body, some foods have the opposite effect as you would think. For example, lemons are acidic, but once broken down by the body, they have an alkaline effect.

Consume Less Acidic Foods

Some common acidic foods: carbonated water and club soda, cream cheese, pastries, pasta, cheese, black tea, coffee, beer, wine, pickles, chocolate, vinegar, pistachios, beef, white bread, peanuts, and wheat.

Consume More Alkaline Foods:

Some common alkaline foods: lemon, lime, green tea, onion, kale, asparagus, spinach, broccoli, artichoke, Brussel sprouts, cabbage, cauliflower, cucumber, sea vegetables, collard greens, sweet potato, lettuce, celery, mango, papaya, figs, dates, melons, grapes, kiwi, pear, beets, blueberries, mushrooms, soy beans.

Look at all the **GREEN foods** listed in the alkaline list! Over and over again, you are learning how very important it is to get the green foods in daily. Remember, try to get some in raw and some cooked every day.

For Disease Prevention:

- Buy fresh, then frozen, canned as a last resort
- Buy local when possible
- Minimally processed   (no added sugar, artificial ingredients, trans-fats, excess salt)
- The fewer ingredients, the better

Essential Oils and Disease Prevention and Disease Management:

Essential Oils will be a topic later in the book, but worth mentioning here. There are many "blends" of essential oils that help with illness. For example, to help with mental focus and clarity, there are blends containing a mixture of frankincense, myrrh, lavender and peppermint. Certain blends are helpful for headaches, nausea, congestion, etc.

DAY 2:
HEALTHFUL TEAS, SUPER SPICES AND MORE

Teas are so good for you.
They are truly medicinal!

Green Teas:	Green teas are less processed, therefore contain a little higher antioxidant level that black teas. Benefits: metabolism boosting, help fight Alzheimer's disease and aging.
Matcha Tea	Helps rid body of toxins. Antioxidant rich, Immune Boosting
Sencha Tea	Contains antioxidants and polyphenols that neutralize free radicals
Jasmine Tea	Antioxidant/Weight Loss. Combine with green tea for powerful blend!
White Tea	Reduces stress. Helps prevent storage of fat. High antioxidant value!
Rooibos Tea	Caffeine free and helps with insomnia. Is a very powerful antioxidant tea. It assists with stomach issues and is a weight loss aid.
Oolong Tea	Helps prevent fat from being absorbed.
Pu-erh Tea	A fermented tea that helps shrink fat cells.
Black Tea	Has more caffeine than other teas. Antioxidant. Combats viruses, may prevent cancers and diabetes. Reduces inflammation.
Ginger Tea	Anti-inflammatory, eases arthritis pain, lowers cholesterol
Yerba Mate Tea	Mood boosting. Uplifting.
Darjeeling Tea	May prevent or slow cancers of stomach, prostrate, breast and colon.
Earl Grey Tea	Boosts immune system. Helps fight colds and flu virus. Other benefits: digestive aid, elevates mood, helps prevent cancer and heart disease.
Chai Tea	Contains many antioxidants which help reduce inflammation.
Hibiscus Tea	Helps reduce high blood pressure.
Dandelion Tea	Helps reduce high blood pressure.
Chickweed Tea	Helps with bloating.
Bilberry Tea	Helps curb cravings.
Chamomile Tea	A sleep aid; assists with nervousness and pain.
Mulberry Tea	Antioxidant and aids with weight loss.

Tips on Teas:

- Drink warm tea after meals.
- Once every few weeks, when doing grocery shopping, try a new type of tea.
- Some teas give you energy, so have those early in the day.
- Some teas help you to relax and sleep, so have those types in the late evening.

Super Spices and More:

Experiment with the **SUPER SPICES:** cinnamon, thyme, leaf oregano, red pepper, ginger, turmeric (curry) rosemary, cloves, cumin, nutmeg, coriander, paprika, allspice, black pepper and sea salt. (sea salt that has healthy trace minerals will be gray, beige, or pink …not white)

Learn to cook with these health boosting spices!

Turmeric (curry): helps arthritis and reduces Alzheimer risk. You can use curry in meat marinades, put in chickpea salads, or veggies. Purchase mild curry if you're not a huge fan of the flavor, or take in supplement form!

Paprika and Cayenne Pepper: lowers blood pressure and improves circulation. Use in any vegetable dishes or soups.

Cinnamon is wonderful for diabetics. It helps stabilize blood sugars and minimizes sugar highs and lows. You can use it in overnight oats, smoothies, or applesauce!

Black Pepper: guards against cancer.

Rosemary: It improves learning and helps with focus. It also eliminates or minimizes food borne carcinogens. Try making a paste of rosemary, mustard, sea salt, garlic and rub on meat as a marinade.

Ginger: lowers blood pressure, helps with arthritis pain, and decreases cancer risk. (try ginger & lemon tea)

More healthy food side- kicks:

- **Hot sauce:** helps with curbing appetite!
- **Extracts:** Vanilla, almond, peppermint, maple, coconut, cocoa powder
- **Salad dressings** (yogurt based is good or look for healthier options with the produce in your grocery store)
- Organic **Sour cream, yogurt, cottage cheese.**
- **Mayonnaise:** Olive Oil Mayo or Organic

- **Mustards:** Dijon or regular
- **Organic Ketchup:** the lycopene in ketchup lowers risk of cardiovascular disease
- **Honey:** Get local honey! It fights aging. Dark raw honey or blueberry honey contains the most antioxidants.
- **Juices:** Tomato, V8, Lemon, Lime, Pomegranate, Tart Cherry, Super Fruit Blends
- **Vinegars:** use in dressings and marinades.
- **Horseradish:** detoxifies the body and increases liver's ability to detoxify carcinogens. Try combining with ketchup for dips or spreads.
- **Eat daily:** onion, garlic, berries, mushrooms, cherries, nuts and seeds, greens, beans, pomegranate, superfoods, antioxidants, teas, omega 3's.
- **Herbs:** basil, oregano, tarragon, thyme, rosemary, marjoram, dill, chives, sage, bay leaves
- **Extra Virgin Olive Oil:** keeps brain cells healthy and boosts long term memory. Make a dip with garlic, salt, vinegar, lemon juice and your favorite herbs. Cooking tip: put the FOOD in the olive oil, and then put it in the pan. If you heat the oil first, some of the benefits will be destroyed.
- Every day, mix and drink a mixture of **raw honey, organic apple cider vinegar and cinnamon.** (1 tbsp. of apple cider vinegar, 1 tbsp. honey, and 1/2 tsp. cinnamon.) This will aid in digestion and boost metabolism!

DAY 3:
FEED YOUR SOUL-NURTURE YOUR SPIRIT

Your Higher Power

Most of us acknowledge that there is a higher power. You are truly never alone. Whatever this "higher power" means to you, it is a constant **support and comfort**. It is that inner voice that guides you. Consider joining a church or social group. The support and unity of belonging provides great peace.

Our emotions need attention and nurturing. Your mind needs to be renewed and refreshed daily. Just like your physical body needs exercise, your mind needs spiritual exercise daily.

Ways to achieve being in tune with your higher power:

- A daily motivational, inspirational email that you sign up for
- A book of daily readings or devotions
- Prayer
- Journaling or other writing
- Getting out in nature
- Calming practices such as meditation, yoga, progressive relaxation, guided imagery.

> *"You either get bitter or you get better.*
> *It's that simple.*
> *You either take what has been dealt to you*
> *and allow it to make you a better person,*
> *or you allow it to tear you down.*
> *The choice does not belong to fate, it belongs to you".*
>
> —Josh Shipp

Some Thoughts to Nurture Your Spirit:

1. Attempt to live at **peace** with everyone. Be willing to **forgive** those who hurt you. **Forgive yourself** for any mistakes or wrong doings that you have done. Strive to develop an attitude of faith in God and develop an atmosphere of peace in your life. Forgiveness is necessary to be able to rise above your circumstances.

2. Several times each day, stop for a few moments and pray or meditate. Add some **deep, slow breaths** to the moments of silence. Enjoy the calm and renewal that you will feel. Allowing time for your mind to become clear and peaceful is necessary in order to shut out distractions. During this quiet time, you will find that you can have clarity to solutions you are seeking for problems and for ideas to surface. We all need that time to just "be". Answers to our problems can never come if we are not "still" enough to allow them to.

3. **Learn to listen to that "inner voice"** that you have inside you. Trust your instincts and let them guide you. Put your emotions aside before making big decisions. Wait for that feeling of peace before moving forward.

4. **Listen for God's voice** to lead you when you are at a crossroads and making changes in your life. Strive to make God's way, your way.

5. Remember that **you become the company that you keep.** Surround yourself with positive people and people that want the best for you.

6. Take a few minutes every day to **be thankful** for what you have. Don't focus on what you do not have. Have an attitude of gratitude. Focus on the things that make you happy, instead of the ones that make you sad. Be thankful for what you do have, instead of dwelling on what you do not have.

7. You will be rewarded for all the **good deeds** that you do in secret. Make it your mission every day to make someone's day.

8. **Follow your bliss. Answer these questions.**

    - What do you love to do so much that you lose track of time when you are doing it?
    - What are you good at?
    - What comes easy to you?
    - What are people always complimenting you about?

    Really reflect on the answers to the prompts above. **This is your gift!** In this lies your calling! If at all possible, whatever this "thing" is for you…. make it your life's work. If that is not possible, then at least find more time to spend in this area.

9. **Share your skills and talents with others.** Take advantage of the opportunities you have to do something good. The more you reach out to others, the more God will reach out to you. You reap the rewards when you give of your time, energy, and resources. When you seek to make other people happier, you will be happier yourself.

10. **Think before you speak.** It only takes a moment for unkind words to come out of your mouth. Unfortunately, those words said in anger can have a lasting imprint on another person. Words cannot be taken back. Saying, "I'm sorry" does not take the pain and negative impact away.

11. **Take time in prayer and ask for God to open the right doors and close the wrong doors leading you in the path that is meant for you.** Remember that life involves constant change. Attempt to embrace it instead of fear it. Sometimes in life if you keep hitting roadblocks, maybe you're going down the wrong path. We sometimes get angry when we think God isn't answering our prayer how we want Him to…but in time we'll see what His plan was for us.

12. Take time to analyze **how you spend your time. Who do you give your time to?** What activities take up your time? You can never get your time back. Do you devote enough time and energy to your loved ones?

13. **You can only control yourself.** Don't let mean spirited people get you down. Don't stoop to their level with their negative words and actions. You cannot control their actions, but you can refuse to let them upset you. You cannot control what anyone else will do or say, but you CAN control how you react to it.

14. Life is not fair and it seems that bad things happen to good people sometimes, but have peace in the knowledge that in the end, **God will see that there is justice.**

15. **God offers second chances. Make today a new beginning for you.** Seek guidance and help if you are going through a rough time. There are good people in this world who want to be there for you. The first step is simply to acknowledge that you have a problem and to ask for help.

16. **Let go** of resentment and regret so that you can reduce the suffering and anguish that you might feel. Negativity will sabotage your success and ability to move forward. Give yourself a clean slate and begin a new, better version of you, today!

"Regrets are the tears of choices not made and of good deeds left undone".

-Jonathan Lockwood Huie

"I can't go back to yesterday – because I was a different person then."

-Lewis Carroll

"Real integrity is doing the right thing, knowing that nobody's going to know whether you did it or not.

-Oprah Winfrey

DAY 4: CALMING PRACTICES TO FEED THE SOUL

Breathing   Yoga   Meditation   Guided Imagery
Progressive Relaxation

We have focused on exercising in terms of your physical health. Your heart and lungs will benefit from cardio workouts and your muscles and bones will greatly benefit from strengthening movements. Keep those going in your routine. Today, I want you to consider adding some calming activities into your weekly routine as well. (both physical exercise and other forms of relaxation)

Breathing

I want to you practice taking deep cleansing breaths. When you are calm and relaxed, your breathing is slower and deeper. When you are under stress, you tend to breathe more rapidly and more shallowly. Being aware of this will let you control the breathing.

When you feel tense or anxious, remind yourself to take some **slow, deep breaths.** It Immediately will lower your stress level. Breathe in through your nose to a count of 4, hold for about 6 seconds, then breathe out through your mouth to a count of 8. Repeat this 4 times. Relax your tongue behind the upper front teeth during the exercise. Notice during this type of breathing how your **neck and shoulders relax.** Most of us hold our tension in our shoulders.

Practicing deep, cleaning breaths will work to reduce cravings, stress, and even help you fall asleep. Like with anything else, practicing will enhance the effects of this breathing exercise. Do this every day, at least twice a day. It will help to decide WHEN you will practice this. I make a habit of doing this type of breathing when I'm in the shower, when I'm in the car waiting at stop lights and when I'm going to sleep at night.

Yoga

The word yoga literally means union.
*Yoga exists on the premise that the **mind and body** are one.*

You can attend 10 different yoga classes and have 10 unique experiences. I encourage you to find a yoga class or purchase an instructional DVD for home use. Yoga can be a complete relaxation type of practice or involve more body toning and strengthening elements. There are many types of yoga. As you learn the techniques of yoga, you master control of your body and increase your enjoyment and benefits of the practice.

Meditation

There are many different forms of meditation. For example, there is walking meditation or methods using sounds or silence. By focusing on something peaceful (this can be a sound, a word, a prayer, an image, or your breathing) you can tap into your conscious mind and promote calm and healing. Choose a word or sound that begins with an "ah" or "oh" and ends with an "m" or "n". The humming sound at the end causes vibrations that are soothing to the mind and body.

To meditate:

- Sit comfortably with your back straight
- Close your eyes
- Take a breath and say the word you've chosen out loud, emphasizing the humming sound at the end.
- When you come to the end of a breath, take another slow deep breath, concentrating on the breathing.
- When your mind wanders, bring it back to the meditation.

Benefits of Meditation:

The result of meditation is that you begin focusing your mental energy. This will increase your power, enabling you to concentrate better, perform better, and you are more able to accomplish more in all areas of your life. The time you need this the most is when you feel you don't have time for it! Even just a few minutes a day will have benefits. When you pay attention to something (food, sex, music, art, massage, walking) you will enjoy it more fully. You will feel calmer and more peaceful. You will experience a greater sense of well-being. You can access your inner wisdom more easily. Because your mind is quieter and calmer, you can more easily hear your still, small voice within you and access your inner wisdom. Choices and decisions become clearer to you. Oprah Winfrey said, "Listen to the whisper before it becomes a scream". Sometimes in the clutter and craziness of our day, we are too overwhelmed to make clear, calm, and wise decisions.

Meditation has been shown to:

- Lower blood pressure
- Lower heart rate and respiration rate
- Reduce anxiety, anger, hostility and mild to moderate depression
- Alleviate insomnia, PMS, hot flashes and infertility
- Relieve some types of pain, but most notably, tension headaches

Progressive Relaxation

With progressive relaxation, you will alternately tighten and relax different muscles and body parts, focusing on how it FEELS to relax them. This practice will allow you to unwind, relax and quiet your mind and body. To get the general idea, read the directions below. To be able to be effective though, purchase a CD of progressive relaxation so that you can keep your eyes shut and really relax.

Directions:

Sit in a chair with your legs uncrossed. Hold your hands loosely in your lap. Shut your eyes. If you are ready to go to sleep or wish to take a nap, lie down in bed with your arms loosely at your sides instead of sitting up.

Take a few deep, slow breaths. Breathe in to a count of 4, hold it for about 6 seconds, and exhale through your mouth slowly to a count of 8. Do this four times.

Next, squeeze your eyelids tightly. Hold it for a count of 8. Release your shoulders. Notice the difference between how the tension feels versus how the relaxation feels.

Take another slow, deep breath, inhaling through the nose and then exhaling slowly through the mouth.

Shrug your shoulders tightly and hold for 8 seconds. Release and take a deep breath in, again inhaling through the nose and then exhaling slowly through the mouth…. notice the difference between the tightening of the muscles and the relaxation.

Hold your stomach muscles in tightly for 8 seconds. Release and take a deep breath.

Squeeze your quads (thigh) muscles and hold for 8 seconds. Release and take a deep breath, remembering to exhale slowly through the mouth.

Tighten your calf muscles and hold for 8 seconds. Release and take a slow deep breath.

Tighten/curl your toes. Hold for 8 seconds and then take another slow deep breath.

You can do these exercises just about anywhere. You can do it sitting at your desk at work, in a doctor's office, waiting at an airport or as you are drifting off to sleep.

Make a conscious effort to do this several times a day. You will be amazed at how much less stress and tension you will carry with you. Adjustments can be made to this scenario to do this in bed at night to relax and fall asleep. Give it a try.

Guided Imagery

Guided imagery is a little more involved that the progressive relaxation. It is an exercise in healing and de-stressing. You are led through an experience using your senses (you use your imagination to see, hear, feel, smell and almost even taste what you are picturing in your mind.) Positive images help you relax and can be used to help pain or alleviate fear. It can decrease your heart rate and help with insomnia. It can decrease headaches and improve the quality of life for those who must learn to manage and live with pain. This technique must be practiced so that you can call upon it and use it when you need it.

When I am really stressed (like at the dentist), I do a guided imagery activity where I visualize being at the beach. I focus on the sound of the seagulls, the roar of the ocean waves beating against the rocks, the smell of the salt in the air, and the feel of the ocean breeze blowing my hair. In my mind, I go to a different place (or I might jump out of the window…. I've seriously considered that while sitting in that dentist's chair!)

Tips for maximum effectiveness of calming practices:

1. Remember to pay attention to your breath. Breathe in deeply through your nose and exhale through your mouth

2. Pay attention to the difference in how it feels to tighten a muscle and to relax it.

3. Consider playing soothing music quietly in the background at work, home, or school.

4. Buy CD's of guided imagery exercises, progressive relaxation and/or calming meditative music. Listen to it when you go to sleep or any time that you want to de-stress and unwind. These practices help with pain management and stress.

5. Purchase a DVD of Yoga or find a class that you enjoy.

6. Read the poem, *Slow Dance* on page 111 as a reminder to slow down and enjoy life. Remember to breathe, treat yourself well and surround yourself with positivity, peace and joy.

Nature:

Try to get out in nature at least 10 minutes every day. Even in cold weather, try to get a breath of fresh air and a quick walk outside. Walk in a park type of setting if you can. Instead of listening to music while you walk, pay attention to the sounds and sights. Sit on a bench for a few minutes and watch the clouds as they slowly move in the sky.

"Life is full of beauty. Notice it. Notice the bumble bee, the small child and the smiling faces. Smell the rain and feel the wind. Live your life to the fullest potential, and fight for your dreams."

–Ashley Smith

SLOW DANCE

Have you ever watched kids on the merry-go-round?

Or listened to the rain slapping on the ground?

Ever followed a butterfly's erratic flight?

Or gazed at the sun into the fading night?

You better slow down.

Don't dance so fast.

Time is short. The music won't last.

Do you run through each day on the fly?

When you ask, "how are you?" Do you hear the reply?

When the day is done, do you lie in your bed

With the next hundred chores running through your head?

You'd better slow down.

Don't dance so fast.

Time is short.

The music won't last.

Ever told your child, we'll do it tomorrow?

And in your haste, not see his sorrow?

Ever lost touch, let a good friendship die?

Cause you never had time to call and say, "Hi"?

You'd better slow down.

Don't dance so fast.

Time is short.

The music won't last.

When you run so fast to get somewhere you miss half the fun of getting there.

When you worry and hurry throughout your day,

it is like an unopened gift….thrown away.

Life is not a race, do take it slower

Hear the music, before the song is over.

- Author Unknown

DAY 5:
ANTI-AGING

Aging is a bad word in our society. We all want to look and feel younger! There are many "secrets" to aging well. Are your choices making you older or younger than your biological age?

Visit this website and calculate your "real age". www.realage.com

This will be an eye opener for you. It will make you more conscious of the types of life stressors that contribute to your longevity. Our choices have a direct effect of on "real age". What is your "real age"? _____

Look Younger! Focus on the Skin

How your skin ages:

As we age, cell renewal slows down: new cells aren't produced as quickly and old ones hang on longer. Cell membranes become damaged and fail to function as well as they used to. Free radicals and stress attack your skin (pollution, stress, cigarette smoke, sun, disease, lack of amino acids and healthy fats, etc.). Your skin becomes dry and estrogen production and thyroid function slow down.

Tips to Minimize the Signs of Aging on your SKIN and BRAIN!

1. Cover up. Use **sunscreen!**
2. **Use a good moisturizer twice a day to say hello to the glow!**
3. **Stay out of the sun** as much as you can. Use protective clothing when in the sun.
4. Get adequate **sleep to** let those skin cells **regenerate!**
5. **Nightly routine: wash** your face well and **remove make up.**
6. **Spritz your face** with water or a commercial facial hydrating spray several times a day.
7. **Drink more water** (keeps skin elastic and supple and helps brain function)
8. **Don't drink through straws.** It causes wrinkling around the mouth.

9. See a **dermatologist** once a year to get skin checked for irregularities.

10. **De-Stress!** Learn stress reduction techniques.

11. Do **cardio exercise!** (skin and brain receive more oxygen and nutrients)

12. Try **yoga** (stretching and firming)

13. Consume blends of **antioxidants and phytochemicals daily.** Good sources include apricots, cantaloupe, lemons, pecans, almonds, sunflower seeds, olive oil, coconut oil, leafy greens, whole grains, nuts, fruit, fish, red wine or grape juice, tomatoes, healthy fats, dark chocolate, pineapple, tomato paste.

14. Drink **green and white tea!** (powerful antioxidant)

15. EAT **high water content foods** so that the water is absorbed better! leafy greens, melons, tomatoes, eggplant, squash, cucumber, lemon, radishes, strawberries, celery, iceberg lettuce, zucchini, apricot, blueberry, oranges, peaches, pineapple, plum, raspberry.

16. **Consume healthy fats and omega 3's:** cold water fish, wild salmon, fish oil, cod liver oil, algae supplements, fiber, peas, beans, fruits, vegetables, vitamin C rich foods such as berries, bell peppers, and citrus fruit.

17. **Other foods** that assist in anti-aging: Olives, dark potatoes (red and purple), variety of colorful fruits and vegetables, salmon, halibut, sardines, tuna, trout, walnuts, cod liver oil, flax seed oil, dark chocolate, avocado, nuts and seeds.

18. **Stay connected with other people.** Plan meals and activities with others. Have a support system.

19. If you live **alone, get a pet!** Pet owners are happier and live longer!

20. Do activities like **games and puzzles** to keep your brain functioning sharp. Challenging your mind will keep it working well.

21. **Eliminate refined sugars and flour and processed foods** (white bread, pasta, potatoes, pastries, pie, cookies, cake, foods in a box, prepackaged foods)

22. **Do all you can in your home to clean the air.** (plants, filters, house plants).

Wrinkle fighters!

- Retinol Cream, Vitamin A, Peptides, Vitamin C and Vitamin E , Vitamin B

- AHA's (Alpha Hydroxy Acid), Glycolic Acid, Hyaluronic acid

- 100% argon oil or organic coconut oil for skin, hair and nails.

- Use ammonia free hair dye.

- Supplement – (phytoceramides) 350 mg daily (hydrates skin from inside out)

Teeth whitening!

- A **white smile** takes years off your look. Mix a small amount of toothpaste, baking soda and hydrogen peroxide and brush with this mixture once a week to eliminate stains and keep teeth white.

- Try **coconut pulling** (swish 1 tablespoon in your mouth for 15 minutes once weekly). This reduces bacteria, plaque, gingivitis, and whitens teeth.

Go Organic with Skin and Body Products

It is wise to use organic products (cosmetics, hair care, deodorant, cleansing items, lotions, toothpaste). Organic skin care is the smartest way to clean, treat and condition your skin without using harmful toxins (petroleum's, preservatives, artificial dyes and colors).

What you put on your skin enters your body and bloodstream! In a warm bath or shower your skin pores open and take in the chemicals in our products we use as well as the toxins in the water itself. For this reason, you should buy a shower head with a filter.

Embrace Aging:

Aging is a privilege. Let's strive to be thankful for every day that we wake up. There are many things we can do to help us to age well. Live well and live long.

DAY 6: STRESS LESS

Worry   Anxiety   Uneasiness   Anguish   Fear   Depression   Panic

All of us need some skills to help alleviate and manage stress.

I hope that you are practicing the early morning journal routine that we learned about already. Simply writing down your concerns, fears, worries, issues is the first step to dealing with them. After writing them down, cross out the items that are not in your control. Focus on the ones you can come up with a solution for. Pray and let go of the things you cannot fix, control or change. Remember that the reason to focus on the negative things early in the day is so that later at night when you are trying to wind down to rest, you can remain calm and at peace.

Stress is a mental, emotional, or physical tension that you feel in response to stressful situations, people or events. It causes anxiety or uneasiness. If continued and chronic, it will affect your health. Physical exercise is one of the most powerful ways to reduce stress. The relaxation and calming practices we've talked about are great tools too.

Stress is a part of life. Learning to manage your stress is important. The quality of your relationships with friends, family, and co-workers will determine your stress level and in turn your health! The biggest factor that produces stress in our lives is negativity.

In your relationships, do any of these things occur?

- Do you feel "put down" by loved ones? Are you criticized?

- Do you feel guilty, sad, or bad about yourself?

- Do you feel that you are a disappointment to your loved ones; that you do not measure up?

If you said yes to the questions above, you need to evaluate your life and your relationships. Consider making changes that will make you happier and calmer.

Some sources of our daily stress are:

- Financial worries

- Time pressures, over-commitment, deadlines, perfectionism, career

- Relationship issues

- Worrying, fear, negativity, unresolved issues

- Noises, environmental factors

- Illness, depression, anxiety

Directions: Read through this list of stress symptoms.

Checkmark or highlight the issues you have experienced in the past 6 months:

_____ Sleeping problems or changes in sleep patterns   _____ Poor immunity…more frequent colds, etc.

_____ Headaches   _____ Changes in eating patterns

_____ Stomach Ache/Nausea   _____ Feelings of sadness or depression

_____ Chronic Pain   _____ Excessive worrying

_____ Irritability   _____ Intestinal problems

_____ Feeling nervous or having panic attacks   _____ High blood pressure

_____ Illness

This next list will demonstrate how life events add stress to our lives. Checkmark or highlight any of these that have happened to you in the past 18 months:

_____ Death of a family member or close friend

_____ Divorce

_____ Break-up or separation

_____ Vacation

_____ Extended family over for a holiday meal or celebration

_____ Health issue of loved one

_____ Major change in eating habits

_____ Sleeping issues

_____ Change in school or employment

_____ Change in residence

_____ Marriage

_____ Retirement

_____ Personal injury or illness

_____ Marital reconciliation

_____ Pregnancy

_____ Addition to family

_____ Change in financial status

_____ Spouse begins or stops work

_____ Trouble with boss

_____ Change in work hours or conditions

_____ Change in recreational, church or social activities

_____ Legal Issues

_____ Change in the amount or severity of problems with significant other

_____ Addition of a pet to the family

As you can see, even positive life events are listed. Even "good" things such as a vacation or a marriage are stress inducing.

It makes sense that the more you can do to reduce the stress in your life, the healthier you will be. Stress takes a toll on your body. Much disease is stress related. Do what you can to reduce the stress level in your life. Practice good habits to help you deal with the daily stressors we all face. Treat yourself well. Exercise, eat healthy, get a massage, draw, write, color, or paint. Do whatever it is that makes you calm and happy.

The adrenal glands are where hormone production takes place. Under any stress, the body goes into flight or fight mode. The adrenal glands increase production of hormones such as cortisol. Cortisol helps moderate the stress. Cortisol however, causes the thymus gland to shrink. It also leads to belly fat! The thymus gland has the "killer cells" which fight infection and cancer. A weakened immune system makes us more susceptible to getting diseases such as lupus and fibromyalgia.

What are your worries, concerns, stressors, annoyances, problems?

List everything that comes to your mind:

(Remember, this should be a daily practice that you do early in the day, every day!)

_____
_____
_____
_____
_____
_____

Look over your list and mark out the things you have no control over. Then go back and look at the ones remaining and find a solution to make them better. Learn to let go of what you cannot control or fix.

Is there someone in your life with whom you have unresolved issues? In the space below, identify the problem. What are your thoughts and feelings about the situation? As Dr. Phil says, "someone has to be the hero….it might as well be you". Don't let things eat away at you. Don't allow unresolved guilt or negative feelings affect you. Do what you can to resolve it and put it to rest.

_____
_____
_____
_____
_____
_____

Some tips for stress reduction   Less Stress = More HAPPINESS

1. Build a **support system** and ask for help. We all just need a few close friends who we know we can count on. Be a good friend. Nurture your friendships.

2. **Create the reality you want.** Take time to identify what it is you want in your life. Take steps to make it your reality. Decide to be happy.

3. Refuse to let yourself get overcommitted and overextended. **Reclaim some time to do the things you WANT to do.**

4. **Do the right thing.** Even when no one is watching. It will feel really good.

5. Don't let **fear** keep you from achieving things you want. Eliminate negative self-talk.

6. **Enjoy the now.** Focus on the journey.

7. Reconnect with your **passion.**

8. Eat **healthy foods** and take appropriate **supplements.**

9. **Get enough rest.** Get up in time to get ready for your day without feeling rushed. Allow extra time to do things and to get places that you need to be.

10. Drink enough **water!** Many symptoms of illness are due to inadequate water intake.

11. **Take time for yourself!** Find a way to have at least 15 minutes of solitude daily.

12. Try **stress reduction techniques:** progressive muscle relaxation, guided imagery, aromatherapy, affirmations, exercise, sauna, journaling, meditation, hypnosis, music, yoga, spending time in nature, connect with friends…. whatever is relaxing for you.

13. Tackle things one at a time. Make a **"to do" list** and pace yourself.

14. **Learn to say NO. Delegate** some responsibilities to others.

15. **Identify the stressors in your life.** Make a plan to eliminate the stressors that you can eliminate. Deal with things that are in your control.

16. **Live comfortably within your budget.** Use credit cards for emergencies only.

17. **Realize that you cannot control other people.** Their issues, problems and choices are not your battle. You are not responsible for the happiness of others. Use your energy to make good choices for yourself. How others react to those choices is not in your control. Accept loved ones for who they are. Don't waste energy trying to make them into who you want them to be.

18. **Your life is the people in it.** Evaluate the relationships you have with others. Determine if they are healthy or not and if not, plan a course of action to reduce the time you spend with them, if appropriate. Relationships should be a two-way street. If you are always giving but getting nothing in return, you are allowing others to steal your energy and time.

19. **Listen to your instincts.** There are usually "red flags" that you sense when someone is not good for you. You can avoid harmful or stressful situations if you make a conscious effort to listen to your intuition or "gut" feelings.

20. **Simplify and de-clutter your life and space!** Remember, less is more. Get organized so everything has its place. The possessions you have should be useful or meaningful.

21. Take your work seriously, **but don't take yourself too seriously.**

22. **Choose to be happy.** Use positive self-talk. Go through the day looking for the good. I promise you will find it. Use affirmations daily!

23. **Be prepared for the unexpected.** Keep some emergency cash on hand. Keep emergency blankets, water, and food in the car and in your home.

24. **Practice the journaling exercises you've been shown.** It provides focus and direction to your life.

25. **Fitness is your friend.** Find the time! Schedule it on your calendar! Do it!

"The true measure of a man is how he treats someone who can do him absolutely no good".

-Samuel Johnson

"No one is in control of your happiness but you. Therefore, you have the power to change anything about yourself or your life that you want to change."

-Barbara DeAngelis

DAY 7:
BE HAPPY

"Life is what we make it. Always has been, always will be."

- Grandma Moses

Today I want to ask you to be brutally honest with yourself. Answer the questions below. Please put down the first thing that comes to your mind for each one.

On a scale of 1-10 (10 being the highest possible)

1. How satisfied are you with your career right now?
2. How proud of yourself are you in terms of how you are living your life?
3. How well are your needs, goals, desires and dreams being met?
4. How happy are you with the people, things, and situations in your life?

Re-read the questions and think about how you rated them.

What changes could you make in your life so that it would be happier and more satisfying?

It is in your control and power to CHOOSE to be happy. You have a right to be happy.

Realize that you are not responsible or other people's happiness. Also, realize that you ARE in charge and in control of your own happiness!

"Happiness is not something readymade.
It comes from your own actions."
-Dalai Lama

List 3 things you would like to have in your life:

1.._____   2._____   3._____

Now, stop and think. Is it the THING you wanted, or is it the feeling you would have from having it? For example, you probably put money down as one of the things you wanted. But, it is not the money you long for. It is the feeling you would gain from it. You would have financial security.

Happiness doesn't come from stuff. Happiness comes from within. It is a state of mind.

It seems that in our society, we look at the abundance of money and "things" as a measure of success and happiness. I think the longer we live we realize that money and stuff doesn't make us happy. Many of us think we'll be happy when we get the promotion, or the nicer home or better car. We live our lives in the pursuit of happiness, like it is a destination on a map. We spend most of our life waiting to arrive only to realize we missed the whole trip.

Let's slow down and enjoy today and make a conscious effort to live in the now. Enjoy your life and live in the present. One of my biggest regrets is working so very much all the time. I was a single mother of 3 very busy, active children. I wanted them to be able to go to the sports camps and have the latest and greatest clothes and shoes. I worked ALL THE TIME to give them the things I felt they needed and wanted. I wish I would have given them more of my time. That is what kids need and crave. I was so drop dead tired all the time. Half of my life is a blur.

You know, in our "golden years", all the money in the world, the cars, houses, and electronic gadgets won't mean a thing. We will most likely look back at our lives with some regret. Maybe not for the things that we did, but for the things we did not do.

Make time for your family and friends. Don't let time slip away from you. Don't wait for the perfect time to take that vacation, volunteer at the hospital or get a pet. There will never be a perfect time. Don't be so busy working that you forget to make a life. Create special memories in the hearts of those that you love.

What will matter in the end of life is how you lived and loved and the memories you will leave behind in the hearts of the friends and family who love you. What will be your legacy? What will you be remembered for?

"Fill your life with adventures, not things. Have stories to tell, not stuff to show."

-Connie Hughes

"The purpose of our lives is to be happy."

-Dalai Lama

Path to Happiness:

1. Have **integrity** in all areas of your life – in your relationships, with money, with your job, with yourself! Simply be honest about what you want, who you are, what you are or are not willing to do. Give yourself permission to say no to others when you are asked to do something out of your comfort zone or when you feel overwhelmed.

2. Be accountable. Accept responsibility. Without **ownership,** you have no power.

3. Be **committed.** When deciding to do something, move heaven and earth to make it happen   No whining: No excuses. Be an adult.

4. Take **Action.** Remember life is not going to hand you what you want on a a silver spoon. Identify what you want and take small steps daily to get there. Set goals and make it happen. Give tasks 100% of your effort.

5. Get outside and take a happiness break. Look around you. Get out in **nature** and sunshine. Enjoy the view. Sunshine is the best source of Vitamin D.

6. **Eliminate** irritations! They add up and make you sick, tired, miserable, and unhappy! Ask yourself what things and what people are in your life that cause "dis-ease" and distress? What are the energy drainers in your life? What can you do to eliminate or reduce that?

7. Spend some time really evaluating what you feel your **purpose** is. What is your calling? What are you passionate about? What do you want your life to be about? Make sure you have more of whatever that is in your life.

8. In your daily life, be sure to make some time for the things that bring you joy. Make deliberate feel -good choices such as buying yourself flowers, enjoying music, treating yourself to massage or long bath, painting, writing, or reading.

9. You need to have **passion** about your job. If you can't learn to enjoy your job, you need to change careers. You spend too much of your life at "work" not to enjoy it.

10. See each day as a new beginning- a fresh start. Use **affirmations** for inspiration. Smile. Set aside alone time each day. Make someone's day every day.

11. Pay more attention to that **inner voice** and gut feeling that you get at times. Let your conscious guide you and listen to those red flags or bad feelings that you get from a person or a situation. How many times have you looked back at a situation and realized that you should have listened to your inner voice?

12. Your past is behind you. Starting today, you can have a **clean slate.** You are not who you were in the past. You can become who you want to be, starting right now. Be sure to discuss this with the kids in your life. Guide them in setting goals and making decisions. Let them experience consequences of their choices. Don't always bail them out or fix things for them. You want them to make wise choices as adults.

"It's never too late to become what you might have been."

–George Eliot

This is your life. You get to be the writer, producer, director and STAR!

*"I've learned that people will forget what you said,
people will forget what you did,
But people will never forget how you made them feel."*

-Maya Angelou

CHAPTER 5 RECAP:

1. In Day one of this chapter you learned a lot about **disease prevention.** Food truly is medicine. What you learned is to eat **inflammation** fighting foods and to follow an **alkaline diet** to keep your body as healthy as possible.

2. On day two, you read about a variety of **healthful teas.** Many teas have medicinal properties. You also learned a variety of **super spices** to incorporate into your meals. Many other condiments and additives were discussed as well.

3. Day three was about **feeding your soul and nurturing your spirit.** Peace can be found by truly **forgiving yourself and others** for any wrong doing. Learning to focus on your breath is a key factor in maintaining calm in your life. Most of us believe in and rely on **a higher power** for strength and guidance.

4. **Calming practices** to feed the soul was the topic for day 4. Deep cleansing breaths, yoga, meditation, guided imagery, progressive relaxation, and spending time outdoors in nature were all discussed.

5. **Anti-Aging tips** was the subject for day 5. Tips were given to help you age well in terms of your skin and brain health. Other related topics were oral health and body care products.

6. For day 6 the topic was **"Stress Less".** Who doesn't need skill to manage and eliminate stress is our lives? Tips to deal with worry, anxiety, anguish, fear and depression were discussed.

7. **Be Happy!** This is the topic for day 7. You learned that happiness is a state of mind and that you deserve to be happy. Choosing happiness is within your grasp. Many tips to **find happiness** were given.

List some things that you intend to start doing.

_____   _____

_____   _____

_____   _____

_____   _____

List some things that you are going to stop doing.

_____   _____

_____   _____

_____   _____

_____   _____

_____   _____

Identify any roadblocks that you have. What can you do about them? Come up with a plan or solution to your roadblocks.

_____

_____

_____

_____

_____

_____

CHAPTER 6 - WEEK 5

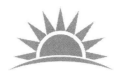

DAY 1:
SOOTHING SLEEP

Sleep is a powerful tool for body renewal. The ideal amount of sleep needed varies from person to person but most adults need 7-8 hours of sleep each night. Sleep allows the body to renew itself, heal, and restore energy. If you are getting adequate sleep, you wake up before the alarm clock goes off and you feel good during the day. It is important to get enough sleep:

Think back to the last time that you were sleep deprived for several days in a row. You probably felt jittery inside and were unable to think or focus.

- Without adequate sleep, you experience a greater chance of injury/accidents.

- Lack of sleep weakens the immune system. (you will be more likely to have colds, flu, any illness or disease).

- Stress is increased by lack of sleep. This will also weaken the immune system.

- Without enough sleep, you will experience confusion, lack of concentration, reduced alertness, and memory loss.

Some tips to promote better sleep

About 1/3 of your life is spent in your bedroom! Do everything you can to make it a relaxing, peaceful, calming and healthy place to be.

1. **Establish a routine** before bedtime. This will signal your brain that it is time to go to sleep.

2. **Consistency is important.** It is best to go to bed about the same time and get up about the same time every day.

3. **Do something positive before going to sleep.** Write in a journal, meditate or pray. Try to clear your mind. Don't dwell on the problems you had that day or worry about your list of things to do for tomorrow. End the day on a positive note.

4. About an hour before going to bed, **reduce the lighting i**n your environment. This will signal to the brain that is time to "quiet" down.

5. **Try to avoid caffeine, nicotine, and alcohol in the evening.** They delay and interrupt sleep patterns.

6. **Don't snack late at night.** Try not to eat for 2 hours before bedtime.

7. **It is best not to exercise 2-3 hours before bed.**

    There is one exception to this. It may be helpful to do a few yoga stretches before bed. Examples are pigeon pose or tree pose. Practice deep breathing at the same time.

8. Do everything you can to effectively **deal with the stress in your life.** Being anxious releases the stress hormones adrenaline and cortisol. They elevate your heart rate and keep you from being able to fall asleep. Make a conscious choice NOT to dwell on things at night.

9. A **warm bath** might help with calming you before sleeping.

10. Make sure your cleansing and **beauty routine is conducive to sleep.** Consider using a lavender scented face wash or body lotion and a mild toothpaste at night. These scents will signal your body to slow down. Certain scents, herbs and spices do the opposite, signaling your body to wake up instead of shut off. Examples of these are peppermint, eucalyptus and rosemary. Avoid those at night.

11. If you have trouble sinking into sleep and shutting your brain off, consider utilizing **progressive relaxation or guided imagery** as you go to sleep. Listening to quiet, soothing music also helps.

12. **Turn off all electronics** about an hour before bed. This will signal to your brain that it is time to begin to turn off.

13. Try natural sleep aids. Alteril works well for me. It has 3 natural agents to help you to fall asleep and sleep soundly. Magnesium, valerian root, or tart cherry juice is also helpful for sleep.

14. Don't watch or read about anything **violent, negative or scary** before bed. Don't work on bills or work projects and hour before bed. Avoid anything intense or worrisome before trying to sleep.

Sleep environment:

1. Green, blue and neutral colors are best for the bedroom.

2. Keep the bedroom as dark as possible. Limit the light that you see. Even a little bit of light from electronics, night lights and alarm clocks is detrimental to sleep. Close the door if you have a hallway light on and consider facing your alarm clock away from you.

3. For optimal sleep, the temperature in your bedroom should be between 60 and 65 degrees. If you tend to get too warm when you sleep, try a cooling gel mattress pad underneath your sheet.

4. It is important to have a consistent sound during sleep. White noise machines really help. Running a ceiling fan or a humidifier is good. Other options to try are listening to audio books or meditation CD's on low as you drift off to sleep.

5. The bedroom should be calm, inviting, and relaxing. Remove all work, magazines, projects, and electronics from your bedroom.

6. Don't listen to the news as you go to sleep. Even if you don't remember it, you dream about the things you focus on before falling asleep. Most of the content in the news is negative. Inform yourself of news events during the day, not before sleep.

7. We love our animals, but they should not be able to sleep in bed with us. Your sleep is very much disturbed by animals. Make your pet a wonderful bed on the floor. You both will sleep more soundly. I have a confession however. Baxter sleeps with his mommy. I have decided that the comfort that I get from him being right there is worth any aggravation. Truthfully, he usually does not wake me up.

DAY 2: SERVING SIZES AND PORTION CONTROL

I know that this is one of my problems and I'm guessing that it is an issue for you as well. I struggle with appropriate servings sizes and portions. Below are some tips to help you. You might begin with measuring things. Then, after a week of two of measuring, you'll be able to make better, more appropriate choices in terms of the amount of foods that you consume.

Serving Sizes:

Fruit — A serving of fruit is ½ cup each of each type of fruit You need 3 or 4 servings daily (vary the color!). Remember your goal of having at least 3 different types of fruit at breakfast and no more fruit after the first half of the day.

Be sure some of the fruit is the whole fruit – raw, in its natural state.

Vegetables — Servings for vegetables is ½ cup to 1 cup of each type

Try to get a total of at least 5 servings daily. Just like with fruits, you want to vary the color to get a variety of health benefits.

Every day, eat some raw and some steamed or cooked.

Grains — A serving of grains, rice or pasta is ½ cup.

Be sure to choose 100% whole grains

Appropriate daily intake is 3 or 4 servings.

Bread — 1 slice of bread is a serving. Be sure the bread is whole wheat. The word "whole" should be listed in the first ingredient. The most nutritious breads will have many types of grains and seeds.

Protein — The quality of the protein you eat is very important. Choose organic lean protein sources and eat a small amount often. Consuming 3-4 ounces of protein 4 or 5 times per day is your goal. A good visual of the amount of protein you should eat at one time is the amount that is the size of your palm or the size of a playing card.

For optimal health, include vegetarian sources of protein and limit animal products.

Dairy — Serving size ½ cup   1 to 2 servings daily

Healthy Fats — A serving size of oils for cooking or salads would be about 1 tablespoon. For nuts/seeds it is about ¼ cup, or what you could fit into the palm of your hand.

Portion Control:

Eat 4-6 small meals throughout the day for optimal health. This will allow your body to metabolize food more effectively. Remember that the combination of foods is important. Always combine a lean protein, healthy fat and complex carbohydrate. You should eat every 3 or 4 hours. Eating often will keep you full and satisfied. We make poor food choices when we are extremely hungry. Use a smaller plate and have appropriate serving sizes.

Do an internet search and take a "portion distortion" quiz.

You will be amazed at how portion sizes have changed over the years. Our idea of an appropriate portion size is much larger than what it should be. This will open your eyes and make you think about those large helpings. The key to getting our waistline where we want is to consume appropriate amounts of food and choose nutritious healthy foods.

Think about the last time you ate at a fancy restaurant. You probably got your meal and thought, "is this all I get"? Yep, that's the appropriate amount of food we should have.

Beware of Advertising Tricks and Gimmicks!

Beware of false claims. Companies hire marketing geniuses. Read the labels for information and don't trust the wording on the outside of a package.

Examples:

1. A fat free food can be loaded with salt and sugar. To make processed food taste good, it will have fat, salt, or sugar. Beware of packaging. Reading the label is the only way to know what is in the product.
2. A food can be labeled "all natural" and be bad for your health.
3. Multigrain bread is mistaken by consumers for healthy food (you want whole WHEAT, not multi-grain).
4. To be truly organic, the label must say "Organic" or even better would be "100% organic". If it says "made with organic" or "organic ingredients", some of the contents are organic, but not all. Buyer beware!
5. A food may be marketed "sugar free", but it could be loaded with fat and salt.
6. Watch for hidden sugar. A manufacturer does not want to list SUGAR as the first ingredient, so on the label they may break the sugars down separately and list 4 or 5 types of sugar. A few examples are sucrose, dextrose, rice syrup, brown sugar, cane sugar, and barley malt.

DAY 3:
HEALTHY EATING WHEN DINING OUT

Most of us eat out a lot. It's what we do to visit with friends and family. Many people have jobs that require lunch meetings as well. The good news is it is possible to eat healthfully when dining out. Most restaurants are getting better about offering lower calorie, healthier options. As mentioned early, be sure to always drink some water and eat some raw vegetables prior to heading out to a restaurant or function where you know there will be lots of temptation. Let's learn some tips to make better choices!

Pay attention to the descriptions of meals on a menu. See below for a guide:

The "Yes" List -choose these!	Just say No!
Baked	Cheesy
Poached	Creamy
Boiled	Fried
Broiled	Battered
Fresh	Crispy
Grilled	Loaded
Light	Stuffed
Multi Grain	
Seasoned	
Stir Fried	
Roasted	
Reduced	

Helpful Hints to Make Healthy Choices when Dining Out

1. Order from the weight watcher, light menu, senior menu, half-size, or lunch size menu.

2. Order a regular meal and split it with a friend (order an additional side salad).

3. Order the larger size meal, but immediately when receiving your meal, ask for a box and pack half of the meal up to take home to eat the next day.

4. Before you leave home – drink a glass of water and eat a piece of fruit or some raw veggies.

5. *Decide what you are going to have before you get to the restaurant.* Don't open the menu and be tempted by all the pictures that make your mouth water!

6. Be the first person at the table to order…so you won't be tempted by other's unhealthy choices.

7. Use a phone app such as "Lose it". You can look up calories and nutrition facts of foods to help you make healthy choices. We sometimes think a soup, appetizer, or salad is a healthier choice, but it may not be! It depends on the ingredients in it as well as how it was prepared.

8. Instead of entrée, order 2 of these: soup/salad/half sandwich.

9. Order a healthy appetizer and salad instead of a meal.

10. Order sweet potato instead of white potato. (try to eliminate white bread, potato, rice or pasta)

11. Ask for less cheese or low fat cheese.

12. Ask for marina sauce instead of Alfredo or creamy sauce.

13. When you order pizza, get thin crust and pile on veggies. Skip the meat. Eat a salad before the pizza and limit serving to 2 slices of pizza.

14. Order lean protein and 3 different veggies for your meal: skinless grilled chicken, grilled fish, eye of round sirloin tip, top round, bottom round, top sirloin, mixed green salad and 2 other NON-white veggies. Cauliflower is the one exception to the non-white vegetable rule. Other great options are asparagus, broccoli, tomatoes, spring vegetable mix, mushrooms, onion, green beans, carrots, squash or zucchini.

15. Eat NAKED food: get any sauces, dressings, toppings on the side…dip fork in it before you put the food on the fork.

16. Eat mindfully and slowly (chew 25 times…put fork down between bites). It takes 20 minutes for the brain to signal that you are full.

17. Whole grains, quinoa, brown rice, whole fruit and veggies are good choices.

18. AVOID: sugar, white bread/pasta/rice, pastries, baked goods, frozen desserts, sweet sauces like barbecue, ketchup, duck sauce, syrup, fruit glazes.

19. Use a smaller plate. This is a good visual trick. You'll feel like you are eating more than you are.

20. Every day, make one of your meals a large salad. The volume of food you can have with all the mixed greens will be very satisfying.

21. Many salad dressings are extremely high in fat and calories. Ask which dressing are lower in calories and fat. Usually vinegar based dressings are good choices. My personal favorite is raspberry vinaigrette.

DAY 4:
SIMPLE FITNESS ASSESSMENTS

It is a good idea to keep track of your progress. As you become more and more fit, you will be able to do more repetitions of a weight or use a larger weight. You'll be able to walk or jog further, or stay with the same distance and work on increasing your speed. Some simple things you can do on your own to evaluate your fitness level and progress are below:

Perform these evaluations once every month or two.

Record it in some way so that you have a visual reminder. You can add your fitness activities to a journal sheet or jot it down on a calendar. Any method that works for you is fine. Don't compare yourself to other people. It is fun and motivating to challenge yourself and see your progress.

1. **Mile walk/run.** Time yourself on a mile run/walk. To be healthy, you want to be able to do a mile in less than 15 minutes. But, for fitness, make it your goal to get it under 12 minutes. Your neighborhood probably has a track that you can go to so you'll have a place to do this. If not, you could map out a mile distance and do your "test" there.

2. **Sit up test.** Challenge yourself for one minute. Count and record how many sit ups you can do in a minute.

3. **Squat Test.** Put a chair against the wall so that it can't move. Stand with your back to the chair seat. To perform one repetition, you will almost sit down but not quite. Your legs and hips will barely touch the seat of the chair, and then stand all the way up. How many can you do in one minute?

4. **Bicep Curl** – What is the heaviest weight you can lift 8 times?

5. **Overhead Press** – What is the heaviest weight you can press overhead 8 times?

6. **Push Ups** – How many push- ups can you do in one minute? You may need to begin by doing push- ups at a wall, or with your knees down on the floor. As you progress, switch to full military style push -ups.

7. Using a bench or a step, how many **step ups** can you do in one minute? For example, step up on the bench with your right foot then left foot, and then step down right foot and then left foot. (up, up, down, down as fast as you can…this is one repetition)

You can make up your own fitness evaluations, depending on what type of fitness activity you are doing or what type of exercise machine or equipment you are using.

DAY 5: NUMBERS TO KNOW

It is a great idea to keep an eye on the numbers below. Calculate the ones that you can and get the others from your doctor or from your next lab results. Keep a file on your lab results and go over all of your numbers once a year. Compare new lab results to the previous year. You are your own best health advocate. Information is power. You need to be on top of your own health information. Your doctor has it on file, but you need to have it and understand it.

_____Weight

_____Height

_____BMI   Goal is 25 or under
                            25-30 is overweight
                            Over 30 is obese
                            Go to WebMd.com to get more information.

_____Waist Size   Goal is 35 or less for women and 40 or less for men

_____Waist to Hip Ratio   Take your waist measurement in inches and divide by your hip measurement in inches.

                                          (Ideal is under .85)

_____Blood pressure   below 120/80 is ideal

_____Cholesterol Ratio   LDL (lousy, low…the lower the better)   Under 100

                                          HDL (high, hero….the higher the better)   Above 50

_____Total Cholesterol   Desirable   less than 200
                                       Borderline high   200-239
                                       High   240 mg and up

_____Blood Sugar   Under 100

_____Triglycerides   Less than 150

_____Target Heart Rate   (60-85% of your maximum heart rate for your age. See WebMD.com)

Information to know:

- Keep an eye on the numbers on the previous page and make a plan with your doctor to get them in desirable ranges. How long you live and how well you live depend on it.

- Don't drink to excess and be tobacco free.

- If you don't have a primary care physician, find one and schedule a checkup. Be sure to get the medical tests that you need. Organize your medical records and choose a friend or family member to be your health advocate. Make a living will. Consider being an organ donor.

- Keep your blood test results on file. On the same piece of paper, record your health information numbers year by year so that you have a record that is easy to review. Doing this will enable you to quickly see any changes.

- Exercise is vital to your health. It is instrumental in getting the numbers on the previous page where they need to be. Schedule your fitness sessions just like you would schedule any other appointment. It is an appointment you need to keep.

- If excess weight is an issue for you, make the decision and commitment to develop a plan to lose the weight! Join a class or a program. Getting your weight in the desirable range will do wonders for your health and your joints will thank you too.

- Eat your way healthy! Eat a variety of colorful fruits and vegetables every day. Eat lean protein and healthy fats. Limit sugar and eat leafy greens daily. Add filtered water to all of that, and you are good to go.

- Stress is a silent killer. Identify your stressors and make a plan to eliminate the ones that you can. Learn stress management techniques to deal with the rest.

- Sleep is important to your overall health. This is when your body can rest, renew and regenerate. Most of us need about 7.5 hours of sleep nightly.

DAY 6: YOUR PHYSICAL ENVIRONMENT

Promoting a healthy environment is so important. You need to do everything you can to make your physical environment pleasing to the eye and more importantly free of toxins. There are many things you can do to make your physical environment better. See how many of these you can incorporate into your life.

Atmosphere (Colors, Scents, Herbs, Flowers)

Feng shui is the ancient Chinese practice of arrangement and placement of things in your environment. The goal is to achieve harmony with the environment. Different areas of the body are related to different areas of your home. The center of your home is related to overall balance.

Use of color is an important aspect of feng shui. Color can have a great effect on your mood and your stress level. Color promotes emotion and attitude. Pay attention to the colors that are in your environment. It can improve your mood and productivity. One tip is to avoid pure white walls, as they invite stress into your home. A few examples follow.

Red: Red is the color of strength, passion, motivation and physical drive

Yellow: Yellow is linked to mental control. It is an optimistic color. Yellow is positive and **uplifting.**

Green: Green is associated with balance and harmony. It is the color of compassion, caring, sharing, and kindness. It is stress-relieving.

Blue: Blue is the calming, cooling, pacifying and comforting color. It promotes relaxation.

Keep these color tips in mind when you decide to redecorate your home!

In addition to painting certain colors on a wall, you can add color with wall hangings, rugs, pillows, curtains, or other accessories.

Flowers add beauty and fragrance to your home. I routinely buy myself flowers when I go grocery shopping. Having bright, colorful flowers makes me smile. Do that for yourself!

Air Quality, Water Purification, Hidden Agers, and Toxins

If you or family members have asthma, allergies, or any respiratory issues, pay special attention to this segment.

Give some thought to the quality of the air in your home!

The EPA says that the air in your home is 2-5 times more contaminated than the air outdoors! Poor air quality can not only be harmful for those with asthma and allergies. It can cause headaches, fatigue, anxiety, aches and pains, depression, and poor concentration. Use quality air and water filters in your home. Add plants to the home.

Benefits of having plants in your home:

Plants are pleasing to the eye, but more importantly, they reduce indoor air pollution and allow more oxygen into the air. Some great plants to have in the home are:

- Ivy (Devils' Ivy, English Ivy, Parlor Ivy)
- Weeping fig
- Purple Heart
- Ficus Plant
- Peace Lily
- African Violet
- Christmas Cactus
- Garlic Vine
- Chinese Evergreen
- Aloe Vera
- Spider Plants
- Mums
- Snake Plant
- Boston Fern
- Philodendron

Watch for the hidden dangers in your home:

When possible, limit your exposure to toxins. Toxins are in the air that we breathe, the food that we eat, the water we drink, and in all personal products and fabrics in our environment. Toxins are substances that interfere with normal cell function. This cellular malfunction is what causes disease.

1. Instead of purchasing plastic water bottles, consider using a filtered pitcher or install a filter on your sink. Besides the fact that you are wasting a lot of money buying all those 24 packs of water, the plastic bottles are an environmental nuisance.

2. Take off shoes at your door. You would be sickened to learn about the germs that you carry into your home from your feet. Tracking in those toxic particles can be avoided. (Same thing with our pet's paws!   ...wipe them off when they come in the house)

3. Use glass or ceramic products in the microwave instead of plastic containers.

4. Mold is horrible for you - use a dehumidifier if you have a damp area of your home. Remember to run the exhaust fan in the bathroom.

5. Dry cleaning – take the bags off clothing items as soon as you bring them home. Don't wear or use the items for a day or two to let the chemicals air out.

6. Clean "GREEN". Remember, clean doesn't have a smell! Instead of using a lot of different chemicals, clean with white vinegar, baking soda, peroxide, or borax. There are many recipes for non-toxic cleaners and laundry detergents online.

7. Open windows! Air out your home for 10 or 15 minutes daily.

8. Use the sun's power. The sun removes moisture which helps to rid of mold and mildew. The sun will break down bad smells. Occasionally, put liter boxes, pet beds, pillows, car seats, etc. in the sun for a few hours.

9. Have green plants in your home to greatly improve the air quality.

10. Consider getting a filter on your shower nozzle. Most city water has many chemicals added. Filtering the water you shower in will help prevent toxins from entering through your skin. Also, before showering, lightly run a dry loofa over your skin to remove toxins. The hot water we shower in opens the pores of your body and allows the toxins in. Therefore, removing them from the surface of the skin before you shower eliminates some of it from getting into the body.

11. Give some thought to an air purification system for the home. You can get attachments for furnace/air conditioning units or free standing units.

12. Discourage tobacco smoking in and around your home.

13. Vacuum and clean carpets, rugs and floors often. When you vacuum, do so slowly so you will raise less dust as you go. Empty the vacuum cleaner bag or compartment outdoors. Consider purchasing a vacuum with a HEPA filter.

14. When remodeling, consider changing to all hardwood flooring. Carpets trap pet dander, heavy metals and allergens. When painting, use low VOC products.

15. Upgrade to better quality furnace filters.

16. Avoid aerosols, commercial air fresheners and scented candles. Using them will put many chemicals into your breathing space.

DAY 7: ALTERNATIVE HEALING MODALITIES

There are many types of alternative healing modalities. Some are more known and utilized in other cultures. Thankfully, they are becoming more mainstream in our society. You may choose to try one or a combination of alternative methods. Investigate the many available choices, including:

Chiropractic   Massage   Aromatherapy   Acupuncture   Homeopathy

Herbal Medicine   Ayurveda   Pranic Healing   Reiki   Polarity

Chiropractic

The Association of Chiropractic Colleges says that "Chiropractic is a health care discipline which focuses on the relationship between structure (primarily the spine) and function (as coordinated by the nervous system) and how that relationship affects the preservation and restoration of health."

Chiropractors may do spinal adjustments, decompression, massage, strength training, electrical stimulation or traction.

Benefits of Chiropractic Medicine:

- Pain relief

- Increase flexibility and range of motion

- Enhance healing and reduce inflammation

- Reduce degeneration and injury risks and enhance joint health

- Increase balance and coordination

Massage

Massage as a healing tool has been in existence for thousands of years. Evidence shows that the more massage you can allow yourself, the better you'll feel. Touch is a natural human reaction to pain and stress. Going to a licensed massage therapist is great, but most of us cannot afford to do that a few times a week. Most cities have workshops that teach you and a partner how to give a massage to each other. A few 15 minute massages per week would be greatly beneficial.

Benefits of Massage:

- Decreases anxiety/promotes relaxation
- Lowers blood pressure
- Increases circulation, lymph flow, and immune function
- Reduces recovery time for injuries or surgery
- Increases concentration
- Promotes better sleep
- Reduces fatigue/increases energy
- Releases endorphins (feel good hormones)
- Provides pain relief from headaches, TMJ, and fibromyalgia
- Provides relief from neck, back and shoulder pain.

Aromatherapy

Aromatherapy uses true essential oils from plants to increase wellness. True aromatherapy is so much more than just a pleasing scent. Aromatherapy is used to ease emotional and physical disease. A blend is customized for each client to work specifically with their body to create mind, body and spirit wellness.

Examples of a few conditions that essential oils can alleviate:

Bronchitis, Anxiety, Insomnia, Depression, Hot Flashes, Muscle Pain, Nausea, Burns, Arthritis, Mental Focus

How to use Aromatherapy:

Ways to use aromatherapy include putting a few drops in a carrier oil like a massage oil, which is then applied to the skin, in bath water; in a diffuser; in a spray mist; or on a tissue or pillow. When I am having sinus issues, I put the stopper in the tub so that water will build up at my feet. I put 5 or 6 drops of eucalyptus oil in the tub. It gets into by body through the pores in my feet and I am also breathing it in as I shower.

For true medicinal purposes, be sure to use the true essential oils, not just the perfumed lotions. Perfumed lotions you purchase at local stores smell good, but have no true medicinal value. Be sure to buy 100% pure essential oils. They are available at health food stores or on-line companies. There are recipes available where you purchase them. You can make blends of essential oils for various health issues.

I recently purchased a Himalayan salt lamp that has a removable container to put essential oils in. I love it! I put peppermint in it if I have a headache. I use lavender later in the day for the calming effect before sleep. These salt lamps are wonderful. I encourage you to purchase one. Any natural foods store will have them or you can find them easily online. They come in many sizes and shapes. They are a natural source of fresh air. The salt lamp cleans and deodorizes the air. They reduce allergy and asthma symptoms and ease coughing.

Frequently Used Oils

1. **Eucalyptus** – good for coughs, colds, bronchitis, and asthma (do not use during an asthma attack). Also, good for sore muscles.

2. **Ylang-Ylang** – Good relaxant, but can also be good antidepressant—it depends on what the body needs; slightly lowers blood pressure.

3. **Geranium** – balances hormones in women; a relaxant and anti-depressant. Balances, stabilizes blood pressure, induces sleep.

4. **Peppermint** – Helps headaches, digestive disorders, nausea, helps wake you up, energizes you, relaxes muscles, and relieves arthritis symptoms.

5. **Lavender** – One of the safest, most relaxing and soothing oils. It is good for treating burns, wounds, and skin problems. It reduces inflammation, headaches, relieves pain through nerve endings, boosts immunity.

6. **Lemon** – Uplifting, also relaxing, helps with focus, good for treating wounds and infections, helps clean out lymphatic system, fevers, sore throats and coughs, reduces inflammation and stiff muscles.

7. **Clary Sage** – It is a natural painkiller. It also balances hormones, relieves depression and insomnia, and rejuvenates adrenal glands. Side effects may include headaches, nightmares, or elevation of blood pressure. To be safe, do not use with disorders involving estrogen levels.

8. **Tea Tree** – Natural anti-fungal, helps boost immune system, stimulates immune system and white blood cells, regenerate scar tissue, reduces swelling.

9. **German Chamomile** – Very relaxing, helps with anxiety, helps with depression, menopause, PMS, inflamed or bruised skin, numbs joint pain, increases white blood cells.

10. **Rosemary** – Mental stimulation and helps boost immune system. Good for muscle aches, improves memory, stimulates nervous system and increases energy, helps lymphatic system, reduces nausea, penetrates muscles and rheumatic pain, lung and sinus congestion. Caution: May increase blood pressure.

Experiment with essential oils and see which ones would benefit you.

Acupuncture

Acupuncture involves the insertion of very fine needles into the body at specific locations. These locations and functions have been studied by the Chinese for thousands of years. This causes the re-activation of the natural flow of energy in the body and restores health. By stimulating the autonomic nervous system, endorphins (the feel-good hormones) are released. Acupuncture can also increase blood circulation, relax muscle spasms, reduce pain and stimulate nerve activity.

Homeopathy

Homeopathic medicine is the second most widely used system of medicine in the world.

It is based on three premises: that like cures like, using minimal doses, and use of a single remedy. It is holistic and treats the cause instead of the symptom of a medical issue. Tinctures are made from plants, minerals and animal venom. Homeopathy is commonly used for fever, cough, flu symptoms, sinus, upper respiratory issues, nausea, indigestion, sleep aid, pain relief, stress, and anxiety.

Advantages of homeopathy are:

It is natural, safe, effective, and non-addictive!

It makes sense to me, to treat the cause of a health issue, rather than mask the symptom with a medication!

There are circumstances, however when medications are necessary.

Herbal Medicine

Botanical Medicine from plants or plant parts

Add these superstar herbs (Nature's Medicine) to your diet weekly!

1. **Ginger:** fights inflammation and is a digestive aid.
2. **Turmeric:** Cancer fighting, anti-inflammatory, cleans and restores
3. **Fenugreek:** reduces cholesterol, anti-inflammation
4. **Cinnamon:** stabilizes blood sugar levels, high antioxidant level
5. **Chamomile:** sooth nerves, digestive aid, cancer fighting
6. **Garlic:** anti-bacterial, anti-viral, anti-fungal, fights disease

Ayurveda

The Science of Life

The goal of Ayurveda is to find imbalances in an individual and offer interventions that will restore the balance. This can be done with diet, aromatherapy, herbs, massage, music, or meditation. Guidelines and suggestions are given on seasonal and daily routines, diet, behavior and proper uses of herbs to attain harmony in body, mind, spirit and environment.

Alternative Healing offers choices of different modalities to heal in a more natural and holistic way. The concept behind energy work is that because humans are a combination of mind, body and spirit, what impacts any one aspect of our creation, impacts all parts. The key to wellness is balance. Energy healing complements traditional medicine. It involves gentle touch and non -touch methods. It offers relief from emotional and physical stress and pain. It is an effective modality for chronic and acute illnesses. It stimulates and strengthens the immune system. A brief overview follows of a few alternative healing modalities.

Pranic Healing

Prana means life-force. In the Old Testament, it is referred to as the breath of life.

Pranic healing is a non-touch, non-invasive form of energy healing that works on the mind, body, and spirit. Pranic Healing is a respected form of energy medicine that is used worldwide. The practitioner scans a person's energy body which consists of the aura and the chakras (energy centers) that are part of the physical, emotional and spiritual energy body. Pranic Healing deviates from traditional western psychology and medicine in that a client does not need to speak about what is troubling them – physically or emotionally. While scanning a client, the practitioner feels energetic "depletions" or "congestions" and works on restoring balance and healing to the whole system.

People who have received Pranic Healing prior to and after surgery have reported experiencing far less or no pain, as well as a more rapid recovery. Many hospitals throughout the country now have energy healers on their staff, including Pranic Healers.

Reiki

Reiki is a Japanese technique used to promote relaxation and to reduce stress. It helps to restore balance in the energy system of an individual by clearing energy blockages that may cause illness. A Reiki practitioner may use a hands-on or hands-off technique. Chakras of the body are used to bring general health, well-being, and to clear the energy pathways of the body.

Polarity Therapy/Energy Medicine

Polarity Therapy is a holistic system of energy medicine. It was developed by Dr. Randolph Stone. The basis of this therapy is the awareness of energy in the body. It uses energetic exercise, nutrition, body work and communication to unblock and balance the body's energy systems.

Benefits of this therapy may be:

- Relaxation

- Preventative health maintenance

- Relief of illness or discomfort

- Release of tension or trauma from the body

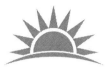

CHAPTER 6 RECAP:

1. On day one of this chapter, you learned how to achieve more **restful, rejuvenating sleep.** You read about how to make your routine and sleeping environment more beneficial and conducive to sound, restorative sleep.

2. Appropriate **serving sizes and portion control** were discussed in day two of this week. Many advertising tricks are used to lure us into choosing different products.

3. It is possible to **eat healthfully when dining out.** Many tips were given in day 3 of this chapter so that you can make more informed, healthful decisions.

4. To challenge yourself, several **simple fitness assessments** were explained in day 4. You can keep a record of some of your cardio, strength, and power abilities.

5. We trust that our doctor keeps a record of our lab results, but we need to be our own health advocate! Different **numbers you should know** were discussed on day 5. I encourage you to keep a file folder of this information from year to year.

6. **Physical Environment** was discussed on day 6. The atmosphere of your home, toxins, air quality and safer ways to clean were all mentioned.

7. Along with traditional medicine, I encourage you to try some of the **alternative healing modalities** you learned about on day 7 of this week. There are so many benefits to them. Give it some thought!

List some things that you intend to start doing.

_____   _____
_____   _____
_____   _____
_____   _____
_____   _____

List some things that you are going to stop doing.

_____   _____
_____   _____
_____   _____
_____   _____
_____   _____

Identify any roadblocks that you have. What can you do about them? Come up with a plan or solution to your roadblocks.

_____
_____
_____
_____
_____
_____

CHAPTER 7 - WEEK 6

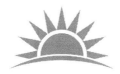

DAY 1: DETOXIFICATION

Toxins interfere with weight gain and diabetes and slow our metabolism. Toxins include anything from environmental pollutants to heavy metals. They interfere with cholesterol metabolism and glucose (contributing to insulin resistance). They cause inflammation, oxidative stress, injury to cells, impaired appetite regulation and altered thyroid metabolism.

Tips and Recommendations for Detoxification:

(Re-boot your system to increase energy, lose weight, cut cravings and enhance your mood).

1. **Eat whole, organic foods.** Consume 8 – 10 servings of colorful fruits and vegetables daily. Organic foods contain at least 2 times the amount of protective antioxidant and anti-inflammatory properties. **Buy as much organic as your budget will allow.** Drink hot lemon water first thing in the morning. Also, eat lime, blueberries, cherries, pomegranate and cranberries.

2. Consume these often: garlic, onions, berries, greens, pomegranate, and drink green tea. Other helpful detoxifying foods are cabbage, pumpkin, seeds (chia, pumpkin, hemp, flax), walnuts, avocado, broccoli, collards, kale, Brussels sprouts, Bok choy, arugula, radish, mustard greens, turnips, turmeric (curry), and organic eggs. Include sea vegetables in your diet! Reminder: an easy way to do this is to buy "green powder" mixes with sea vegetables in it and add it to fruit smoothies or other foods. You don't taste the "greens" this way.

3. More "clean foods" to include each week are cold water fish and free range chicken. Another tip is to do your own bone- brothing with organic meats with bone in them.

4. Filter your drinking water. Purchase a good quality air filter for your home. Remember that adding plants into your home will also help to clean the air.

5. Drink 8-10 glasses of water each day. Drink lemon water, coconut milk, green tea, and herbal teas. Apple cider vinegar (about a tablespoon in a glass of water) before meals aids in detoxification of the body.

6. Cook with healthy oils such as coconut, extra virgin, sesame, and grapeseed.

7. Nourish your digestive system. Remember that most your immune system is in your "gut". Probiotics, flax oil or flax seeds, magnesium citrate, or cod liver oil are good for your digestive system. Other detoxifying supplements are Vitamin C and vitamin C rich foods, lipoic acid, and milk thistle. Try a blend of herbal teas for detoxification. Dandelion root, burdock root, and milk thistle are great together.

8. Take a high quality multi-vitamin/mineral supplement. Check for the recommended daily dosages of B6, B12, folic acid, zinc and selenium. They aid in detoxification.

9. For cleansing the body, sweat **profusely** 3 times per week (far infrared sauna, detox bath, steam room). Take Epsom salts detoxifying baths 3 times per week. (20 minutes).

10. Exercise 5 or 6 times per week for 30-60 minutes each time.

11. Avoid caffeine and nicotine. Eliminate white products (flour, sugar, bread, pasta).

12. **Diagnostic** tests such as hair analysis or saliva tests may be performed to identify what the body has too much or too little of. This is always a great thing to do to rid the body of heavy metals such as mercury, lead, arsenic, and other toxic metals. Check into this if you have an illness or health issue. It is truly miraculous how much better your body can function when it is having the proper balance.

DAY 2: RELATIONSHIPS

You have a relationship with everyone in your life. Your spouse, parents, siblings, co-workers, children, neighbors, and friends are all people you have a relationship with.

One thing that I've learned is that you truly teach people how to treat you. What I mean by that is others learn what you will and will not tolerate or how you will react to events and situations. You tolerate the behavior from someone that mimics what you feel you deserve. This explains why some people in life are called "doormats" and some are called "barracudas".

The relationship you have with yourself is the most important one!

Do you treat yourself as well as you do your family and close friends? Think about the following and see how you are doing in terms of taking care of yourself and putting yourself first. Do you make yourself a priority?

- Do you get enough sleep? Yes No
- Do you get 6-8 hours of exercise each week? Yes No
- Do you schedule a fun activity each week? Yes No
- Do you get at least 15 minutes of quiet/alone time daily? Yes No
- Most of the time do you have good nutritional habits? Yes No
- Would you say that your emotional health is good? Yes No
- Do you feel your stress is under control? Yes No
- Do you feel overwhelmed on a daily basis? Yes No
- Do you spend enough time on fun, recreational hobbies? Yes No
- Can you say no, delegate or ask for help when you need it? Yes No
- Do you feel valued, appreciated, and respected at home? Yes No
- Do you feel valued, appreciated, and respected in the work place? Yes No

Re-read your responses. What areas of your life need attention? Talk to your close friends and family about the things you need to improve on. Ask for help. Make a plan to work on the things you need to do better. Be kind to yourself. Take some of the burden off your shoulders.

The relationship with yourself needs to be healthy so that your other relationships are healthy and positive! Love is not outside you; it is within. The qualities you possess will attract someone with those same qualities. You must love yourself and treat yourself well in order to have a healthy, loving, giving, nurturing relationship with another person.

"Cherish your human connection – your relationships with friends and family."

-Barbara Bush

Our Friends and Family

We need a few close, wonderful friends we know we can count on. They make us feel included, connected, valued, understood, appreciated and loved. We all need a few people that we know we can depend on. To have a friend, you need to be a friend. Take the focus off of yourself and do for others. Go out of your way to be helpful and kind. The rewards will come back to you tenfold!

We are born into our families, but we can CHOOSE wonderful friends who become our family. Choose well and nurture your friendships.

Who are the people in your life that you seek approval, love, appreciation or respect from? Who are the people in your life that you seek to make smile and do nice things for? Name them below:

_____   _____

_____   _____

_____   _____

The people that you identified above are the people that you want to give your time, attention, and devotion to. Surround yourself with caring, kind, and positive people who truly want the best for you. Nurture the relationships in your life. Support and encourage your loved ones. Be attentive and really listen to others. Show gratitude and choose your words wisely. Stay connected to them and give of your time. Schedule time on a regular basis for these loved ones! Don't be so busy making a living that you don't make a life. Make wonderful memories and begin new traditions.

"People do not care how much you know until they know how much you care."

-John C. Maxwell

Personal Note:

I truly delight in being able to do things for my children, Megan, Molly, and Matt. I now also have four grandchildren, Gage, Jake, Macie, and Owen. They are the light of my life and bring more joy to me than I can possibly express in words. You don't know the meaning of "unconditional love" until you become a parent. Molly Cannon, my college roommate and dear friend said something profound that stuck with me. She said "you can only be as happy as your saddest child". Wow. That speaks volumes. It is so true.

Let's make sure that we make time for our loved ones. Give our support and encouragement. Let's make sure that they know with all their heart how much we love and value them. Be present and be involved. That way you will live in the hearts of your family and friends forever.

Relationships

H Have more good times that bad. Focus on the good. Both of you are giving and loving.

E Enjoy each other and make time for each other. Have quality time together yet find balance between your time together and time for friends, family, and yourself!

A Are able to communicate and be heard and supported. Clear, honest, and open communication!

L Live! Laugh! Love!   Make a bucket list and begin to live your dreams.

T Trust…you can trust each other. You should feel at peace, secure, safe and comfortable. Have zero tolerance for physical or verbal abuse.

H Have privacy in the relationship. Make a "date" night each week. Take turns planning it.

Y You take interest in the everyday lives of each other (family, friends, work, and health).

Take time to evaluate all your relationships. Make decisions concerning the time and energy you give to those in your life. Are they fulfilling you or draining you? Hurting you or helping you? Below are the deal breakers! Relationships can be toxic. Evaluate the emotional health of your relationships.

D Does not make time for you.

E Every time THEY need or want something, you are there for them…. but not the other way around.

A Afraid. Do not be involved in a relationship in which you are afraid of someone or their temper.

L Lies. Deceitful people who mislead you or lie to you are not healthy for you.

B Beware of anyone who is capable of pushing, grabbing, hitting, punching, or throwing things in anger.

R Relationship involves control or manipulation of you. (control of the money, time, car, bills, things, or people that you can spend time with).

E Encourages you to do things you do not want to do or that are unsafe, unhealthy, illegal, or dangerous.

A Allows or initiates ridicule, name-calling, or disrespectful tone of voice and behavior.

K Kind of makes you feel bad about yourself. The opposite of up-lifting and encouraging.

E Exhibits evil. Watch how they treat their family members, animals, the elderly, a waitress…. you can tell a lot about someone by observing this.

R Really selfish. It is all about them. You are constantly "giving" and not "getting". Does not listen to you, support you, or encourage you.

DAY 3: INDIVIDUALIZE YOUR PLAN

No two people are alike.

Our health issues, preferences, medications and interests are all different.

Food: Our food preferences are different. I could tell you all day about the benefits of broccoli. But if you hate broccoli, I won't convince you to eat it. You would need to find other greens to add into your diet. I might suggest that you eat grapefruit, but if you are on certain medications, you are told not to eat it. So, you see everyone's issues, likes, and illnesses are different. What is good for one person is not at all for another. I've given you a lot of wonderful information and suggestions about food, but you will need to tweak it to make it be specific for your life.

Fitness: Your fitness plan is also very individualized. The key here is to find movements and activities that are FUN for you. If you do things you enjoy, you will stick with it. I could tell you how wonderful my Pump RX class is and encourage you to come. But, if you hate fitness classes and don't like to exercise in front of others or at a gym, this would not be for you. Maybe you are self-motivated and will do fitness DVD's at home. Maybe you've enlisted a walking buddy and you walk 3 miles 5 days a week. Find what works for you!

Spirituality and Religion are different for everyone as well. You may be comfortable with traditional religion and go to church twice a week every week. That doesn't necessarily mean you are more spiritual than the next person. Maybe you don't go to church, but you meditate and pray and live a life of service. You strive to bring joy to the people in your life. Spirituality is expressed in different ways. Whatever you do, whatever you believe, the key is that you are a light in the world in some way. Teach what you know. Pay it forward. Get involved.

Environment: We all have unique living conditions and family situations. Whatever those are for you, strive to be present. Be in the now. Put electronics down and focus on the people in your life. You will never regret time spent with loved ones. Surround yourself with people who support and encourage you. Surround yourself with positivity. Make your environment pleasing and positive as well. Try to simplify and de-clutter your environment. Everything in your life should be useful, meaningful, or bring joy to you. Eliminate toxins in your environment. Clean air, pure water, and cleaning with non-toxic cleaners are the basics.

Mindset: Daily practices such as journaling, reading, drawing, listening to music…whatever it is that brings you comfort and joy…do more of that! Do what you can to eliminate stress. Use affirmations and positive self-talk. Be as good to yourself as you would your best friend. Schedule "down time". Call a time out every now and then so you can get a mental break.

Blood Type: I strongly encourage you to investigate the recommendations for your blood type. Dr. Peter J. D'Adamo states, "Your blood type is the key that unlocks the door to mysteries of health, disease, longevity, physical vitality, and emotional strength". Based on your blood type, there are certain foods you should eat more of, some to eat in moderation, and some to avoid. Specific types of exercise are better for certain blood types too. There are even recommendations for supplements and teas. I encourage you to read "Eat Right 4 Your Type", by Peter J. D'Adamo or explore Web MD or other online sites for information specific to you.

My son, Matt was going through some health issues several years ago. One of the first things a friend and holistic health practioner did was make recommendations about his blood type. It really opened my eyes about how important it is to feed and nourish your body based on its needs. Matt always wanted to eat what seemed to me like a tremendous amount of protein. But, I learned that based on his blood type, this was good for him.

DAY 4:
FIT FOR LIFE

"We don't stop playing because we grow old: we grow old because we stop playing."

--George Bernard Shaw

As we age, our fitness activities will change as well. As I mentioned earlier, I used to be a runner. This is something my knees just did not want me to keep doing. As I'm aging, I am noticing that I need to limit the jumping types of things that I love to do when I teach my fitness classes. Listen to your body. We will have to roll with the punches and change what we do as we age.

Some tips:

1. As you age, the basics stay the same. The same general rules apply!

    a. Cardio – 30 minutes 5 times per week

    b. Strength- 30 minutes per week

2. What may need to change as you age is the WAY you exercise. Maybe when you were 25 or 30 years old, you liked to jog. Probably at about 35 or 40, you'll find that you need to switch to an activity that will be more kind to your joints. Cycling or swimming are good options as we age. Instead of cardio activities with a lot of jumping, you could switch to water aerobics. There are many types of water aerobics classes. Some are designed to minimize arthritis or joint pain. Some classes are more intense. Find one that works for you.

3. At any age, the key to being fit is variety. Don't do the same thing 5 times a week. If you mix it up, you'll use more muscles in different ways and be much more fit. One day, go for a long walk. Another day or two, take a water aerobics class, ride an exercise bike at home on a rainy or cold day. Variety!

4. As we get into our 50-s and up, **functional fitness** becomes more important. We want to reduce the chances of falls. We also want to increase our chances of being independent and living on our own. Strength, Balance and Core activities are very important. Work with a trainer or take a class to learn movements that will help you in terms of your strength and balance. It is very important.

5. Combining fitness and socializing is even more important as we age. As we reach retirement age, we are not around people all day like we were in our younger years. Maybe we've lost our significant other. I am in awe of our *Forever Young Classes* at the health and wellness center that I work. Instructor Chris Poe and her participants are supportive and encouraging with one another. The bond and sense of belonging and community that they receive from these classes is so important. They look out for each other outside of class as well as in class.

6. One important tip is that you can work out anywhere! Walking is the most simple and least expensive way to exercise. You can walk in your neighborhood park on indoors in a mall in bad weather. There is no limit to the variety of fitness activities that you can do with little or no equipment.

7. You only get one body. This is where you live! Take care of your body so that you can be healthy as you age. Exercise is the key to being able to age gracefully. You want to be able to take care of yourself and maintain your independence. Be kind to your body and to yourself.

8. Check out what is available in your area. Take advantage of the wonderful programs that are offered at senior centers, churches and hospitals. Get plugged in. Get involved. Volunteer if you are able.

DAY 5:
TIME MANAGEMENT & PRIORITIES

"You live longer once you realize that any time spent being unhappy is wasted."

-Ruth E. Renkl

I hope that you will really take today's discussion to heart. The cost of anything that you say yes to is the time that you donate to do it. You can never get that time back. You may have the "disease to please" as Oprah says. There is not enough time for YOU when you spend so much of your precious time doing things people ask you to do. Evaluate the things that other people want you to do, need you to do, or expect you to do. How many of those things are dragging you down? If it is annoying, irritating, draining and sucking the life force out of you, you need to fix it!

Understand the value of time. Learn to enjoy everything you do, or don't do it!

"The price of anything is the amount of life you exchange for it."

-Henry David Thoreau

A story from my younger life:

As a young new teacher, I felt unable to say no to my principal when he'd ask me to oversee something at our school. Remember, I was a single mother of 3 busy children. I coached both basketball and track at our school, coached softball, coordinated Jump Rope for Heart, ran an all-day Saturday basketball program, and more. Good grief, I was drop dead exhausted every minute of my life. Learn that you truly are in control of your time. Don't let others plan your time for you and expect more of you than you can give at the expense of your own sanity and health.

One day, something happened and I exhibited a little assertiveness for once in my life! I found my backbone! As that young mother of 3 children living in an overwhelmed, overcommitted exhausted state, I hit my breaking point and raised my voice for the first time ever and yelled at my principal! I had gotten a phone call from my daughter's school. She was sick and needed to go home. Luckily for me, it was near the end of my school day and I had my planning period at the end of the day. I went to my principal, explaining the situation and asked to leave. He replied, "just so you make your time up". I was appalled. I turned on my heels, glared at him and responded, "Make my time up? What? My God, I LIVE here!" I was so offended! I spent more time at school than he did! That very day, I realized that I really did not want to continue to be such a "yes, sir" kind of person. I began to limit the amount of MY valuable time that I was willing to give away for free at my own expense.

Learn from my mistakes, and take charge of your time.

The greatest reflection of your values and priorities is what you do with your time.

Of course, you have responsibilities in life. You must work to earn a living. Paying your bills and taking care of yourself and your family is a priority. In a perfect world, you will find a way to make what you are passionate about your life's work. If that is not possible, then find a way to LIKE your work and in your spare time, be sure to spend time doing the things that bring you joy.

I encourage you to write down all your responsibilities you've had to do for the past week. Evaluate them. Make a plan to make this less of a burden for yourself. Which ones were not necessary or important to you? Which ones could you delegate to someone else or eliminate? Remember, your goal is to take back more of your time to do what you want to do and spend more quality time with the people who are important to you.

Make a daily or weekly "to do" list. This will help you with time management. A great help is to look at your list and evaluate it. Which item on your list is the one you are dreading? Do it first and get it over with! You'll sigh a great sigh of relief and feel better about your day. A great time saver is to bundle your chores. How many errands can you do all at the same time and avoid several trips out? Simplify your life as much as you can.

List the roles that you have in your life (parent, driver, cook, spouse, co-worker, daughter, son, laundry person, maid, etc.) For the next 24 hours, I want you to pay close attention to the negative thoughts you are having concerning the "chores" you must do to fulfill the responsibilities of those roles you play. What can you eliminate, delegate, or ask for help with?

An example is below:

Roles:	**Feeling Associated with the Role:**
Mother	*ex: overwhelmed, tired*
Cook, Maid, Driver	
Employee	
Wife	
Scout Leader	
Dog Walker	

Maybe this will help you to reclaim your time!

What helps me to say NO is a little sentence that I've memorized. If you are like me, even when you try to say no, you can get talked into things. Put a stop to it and don't allow the conversation to even happen. When I'm asked to do something that I just don't want to do or don't have time to do, I very nicely just say this; "I'm really sorry…I'd help you if I could but I just absolutely can't do that. My plate is too full". End of conversation. No wiggle room to be talked into something. Give it a try.

DAY 6:
FIND YOUR JOY, PURPOSE AND PASSION

"It's never too late to be what you might have been."

-George Eliot

So many times, we don't recognize our calling in life. Often, we make light of it or don't realize it is our gift. Answer the following questions:

1. What is it that you like to do so much that you lose track of time when you do it?

2. What comes easy to you?

3. What is it that other people ask your advice or help with?

4. What makes you happy?

This is probably your calling or purpose in life! If you can't make it your job that pays the bills, be sure to figure out how to do more of that thing in your spare time. Try to find a way to incorporate that "thing" in your job in some way. Share your gift with others and share what you know. This is your gift to the world.

My daughter Molly comes to mind on this one. Molly is a teacher and a very good one. But, she loves to decorate. Her home is full of amazing things. I literally walk around her house and admire and adore her little touches everywhere. Others often ask her advice and help with decorating and Molly loves to do it.

She brings that magic touch to her 4th grade classroom. It's the cutest school room I've ever seen! Her students are very lucky. She's already told me that when she retires, she is going to spend all her time shopping and decorating. She may have missed her calling. Did you? It is not too late! It's never too late. At age 58, I'm just now doing work that feeds my soul.

Without a life purpose, our life has no direction….no compass.

"The two most important days in your life are the day you are born and the day you find out why."

-Mark Twain

"The only way to do great work is to love what you do."

-Steve Jobs

A feeling of satisfaction with our life and sense of joy and accomplishment can only be reached when we have a clear life purpose or mission. Without setting goals and knowing where we are headed, we aimlessly drift through life. Your life purpose is completely up to you. It is whatever you choose it to be. What does matter is that you let it be the focus of your life and allow it to drive your life. In order to provide satisfaction to you, it needs to involve being of service to others in some way. It is more satisfying and motivating if you focus on others.

> *"How would you want your success to be measured?*
> *Not by the money you made or 'things' you possessed.*
> *By what lasting impact or imprint you made on the people in your life.*
> *Create the highest, grandest vision possible for your life because*
> *you become what you believe."*
>
> -Oprah Winfrey

Oprah also said, **"I've come to believe that each of us has a personal calling that's as unique as a fingerprint and that the best way to succeed is to discover what you love and then find a way to offer it to others in the form of service, working hard, and also allowing the energy of the universe to lead you.**

FINDING YOUR LIFE PURPOSE

What is your personal mission?

You will find your life purpose by following your heart, dreams and passions. You are where you are meant to be when you have a sense of exhilaration and stimulation. You should feel energetic and alive performing your life's work. Think about where you are in your life in the following areas:

- Your work
- Your personal relationships with family and friends
- Your hobbies
- In all the activities that take your time, effort and energy

Ask yourself these questions:

1. What do you really want your life to be about?
2. What are your dreams?
3. What makes you feel invigorated, joyful, and alive?
4. What would you do with your time if finances were not a concern?
5. How does your current job make you feel?
6. Do you feel that you have a positive impact on others?
7. Visualize your life in 5 years….10 years….

What do you want to be doing? Where do you see yourself? What will you have accomplished? Who is in your life? Where will you be living? What experiences will you have had?

Evaluate who you spend your time with and how you spend your time. Are you where you want to be? Or, are you living a life without meaning? What do you want your life to mean? In what ways do you help people? If your life were to end today, how many family and friends would be affected? What have you really done to impact the lives of those around you? Picture your tombstone. Decide on one sentence that you would like to be inscribed on it to describe the kind of person you were. What would you like to be remembered for? The answers to these questions will help guide you in the direction you want to go. Find your purpose. Find something you LOVE to do that will make a difference to someone. Generate happiness and joy for yourself and your loved ones.

> *"The meaning of life is to find your gift.
> The purpose of life is to give it away."*
>
> -Author Unknown

My own personal mission statement and what I hope to instill in others:

I will do everything in my power to be happy, productive, positive, and healthy. I will strive to make myself a priority and to make my family and friends know how much they mean to me through my actions and my words. I will try to make a positive difference in someone's life every single day. I will smile and listen with intent to the loved ones in my life. I will give them my time, my attention and my love. I want to be remembered for the kindness I showed to others. I want to make a difference in the quality of life for the people that I cross paths with.

What is your personal mission statement?

Use mine as an example if you wish to write your own. Write yours below:

_____
_____
_____
_____
_____
_____

Reflect on your mission statement often.

Are you taking steps and putting forth effort toward fulfilling it? What will be your legacy? What do you want to be remembered for?

_____
_____
_____
_____
_____
_____

What lasting impact will your words, kindness and presence have made on others? Live your life in such a way that you will live on in the hearts of everyone who knew you. Do good in your words and deeds. Be a light in the lives of others. Be kind. Give of yourself.

"The purpose of life is a life of purpose".
–Robert Byrne

"Don't die with your music still inside you.
Listen to your intuitive inner voice and find what passion stirs your soul."
-Wayne Dyer

DAY 7: LIFE REVIEW AND REFINING YOUR GOALS

Take a few minutes and reflect on your life. Think about the experiences you have had and be sure to learn from them. Some people tend to repeat the same patterns and mistakes over and over. Acknowledge the life lessons you've had and re-focus your goals. Identify what it is you want for your future happiness, success, and joy.

> *"You are not creating a new you; you are releasing a hidden you. The process is one of self-discovery. The hidden you that wants to emerge is in perfect balance."*
>
> -Deepak Chopra, M.D.

List 3 things you wish you had:

1. _____   2. _____   3._____

Now, go back and look at them again. Is it the "thing" you wanted, or was it the feeling you would receive from it? Joy, peace, comfort, belonging and security are the reasons why we want "things". For example, if you put money down as one of the 3 things you wish you had, it would be so that you would be free of worry and have financial security. Begin to evaluate what you want and why you want it. Happiness doesn't come from things.

Let's dig deep now. Answer the questions honestly. Put down the first thing that comes to your mind.

1. Describe yourself. How do you think others see you? Include 5 adjectives in your description.

_____

_____

_____

2. Who is the most influential person in your life?

_____

_____

_____

3. If you could have one "do over", what would it be?

　

4. If you could change your career, what would you be doing?

　

5. What memories of the past still haunt you? What do you need to let go of?

　

6. What's one thing you know for sure about feeling bliss & joy?

　

7. What do you now know better than you did 5 years ago?

　

8. What is the best thing and the worst thing about the age you are now?

9. What are you allowing to rob you of your joy? What or who is holding you back right now? If you were to fully live your life, what change would you need to make?

_____

_____

_____

10. What is your "gut" telling you about what it is that you are supposed to be doing right now? What is that little voice inside your head telling you in that soft whisper that you have not been listening to? What is missing in your life? What are you tolerating or putting up with?

_____

_____

_____

11. What is one change that you could make in your life to give you more peace? What areas of your life could be upgraded or tweaked to make you calmer and happier?

_____

_____

_____

12. What are you most excited about right now? What do you look forward to?

_____

_____

_____

13. What do you want more of in your life?

_____

_____

_____

14. What do you want less of in your life?

_____

_____

_____

15. What is one thing you wish you had more time to do?

_____

_____

_____

16. What would you like to be acknowledged for in your life? If money were not an issue and you knew you could not fail, what career would you have?

_____

_____

_____

Which of these things need your attention?

- Career, Education or Job Training
- Relationship with a loved one or friend
- Relationship with your higher power
- Relationship with yourself
- Your physical environment
- Your health
- Your emotional well-being
- Stress management
- Quality rest and relaxation
- Financial Situation or Plan for Retirement
- Confidence, Self-Love, and Positivity
- Rest and Relaxation Time
- Addiction Issues or Bad habit
- Other _____

What are you willing to change to really live a life that is satisfying and uplifting?

Ask yourself these questions:

1. What changes do you need to make?
2. What can you do to make things better for you?
3. What are you willing to do about it?

It is in your control…make it happen!

Dream it

Visualize it

Make a plan

Re-invent your life

Look, feel, and live better than ever

Show up for your life - be present in the now

"Every word you speak and every thought you think is an affirmation for your future."
—Cheryl Richardson

"Efforts are not enough without purpose and direction."
—John F. Kennedy

Create your Lifetime Wish List:

"Life is not measured by the number of breaths we take, but by the moments that take our breath away."

-Maya Angelou

List 10 things that you want to do, have, be, or achieve in your lifetime.

1. _____

2. _____

3. _____

4. _____

5. _____

6. _____

7. _____

8. _____

9. _____

10. _____

Don't be a "someday" person. Don't put off the things you want to do. There will never be the perfect time to travel, to get a pet, to volunteer, or to create memories with your loved ones. Don't let excuses get in the way of your joy.

In our final years on earth, we will regret working too much, not spending enough time with our loved ones, not making memories, not traveling, not being adventurous, not taking chances, and not really living life.

What are you waiting on? Choose one of the 10 things on your list above and begin to plan it. Make a goal to do one thing every other year from your wish list.

"Life's journey is not to arrive at the grave safely, in a well-preserved body, but rather to skid in sideways, totally worn out, shouting, holy shit, what a ride'!"

-Mavis Leyrer, age 83

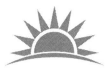

CHAPTER 7 RECAP:

1. In lesson one this week, your focus was on **detoxification.** Removing and eliminating toxins from your water, air and environment are so important to your overall health.

2. **Relationships** were explored in day two of this chapter. The most important relationship you have is with yourself! Many tips were given to maintain healthy, meaningful relationships with the people in your life.

3. On day three, we discussed how important it is to **individualize your healthy lifestyle plan.** Each person is unique. Good choices for you are determined by your preferences, illnesses, medications, limitations, etc.

4. Being **Fit for Life** was the subject matter on day four. As you age, you want to maintain your independence and functionality. The only way to do this is to keep moving! Strength and balance training is vital after age 40. Your task is to find activities that you love to do and stay moving!

5. On Day five, the subject was **time management and responsibilities.** There are only so many hours in the day! You need to do what you can to minimize the time spent doing chores and tasks and carve out quality time for yourself and your loved ones.

6. Finding your **joy, purpose and passion** is so important for living a happy and fulfilling life. Many suggestions were given about this in day 6 of this week's topics.

7. The final new topic of the book is discussed in day 7 of this chapter. You filled out a questionnaire called **Life Review.** Using this tool, you will be able to redefine your goals. Life is short. Take the time to plan and create the life that you want. It is never too late. You can't go back and re-do the past. But, thankfully you can shut the door to the past and make a new beginning today. You can write a new ending. You are the author of your own life story. Make it a great one.

List some things that you intend to start doing.

_____   _____

_____   _____

_____   _____

_____   _____

List some things that you are going to stop doing.

_____ _____

_____ _____

_____ _____

_____ _____

_____ _____

Identify any roadblocks that you have. What can you do about them? Come up with a plan or solution to your roadblocks.

_____

_____

_____

_____

_____

_____

CHAPTER 8 - RESOURCES

HOLISTIC APPROACH TO HEALTH

Being healthy and happy is not a one size fits all kind of thing. You have your own unique health issues, preferences and goals.

A **holistic approach** is best; all things in moderation is a good guide to live by. As you read *Healthy Living by Design,* you incorporated the lifestyle suggestions and habits that worked for you at this time in your life.

We are all a work in progress and our needs and interests evolve and change over time. I encourage you to continue your path to a happier, healthier life. Re-read the book once every year or so, and make more adjustments to your lifestyle as you see fit.

Slowly read the list below. Think about what changes you have made in your life in the following areas:

- Creating a Healthy Physical Environment
- Getting Movement into your Day
- Eating more Healthfully
- Utilizing Calming and Relaxing Practices
- Nurturing your Spirit and Spirituality
- Exploring Alternative Medicine Options
- Practicing Extreme Self-Care
- Having Meaningful Work
- Giving of your Time and Talents
- Nurturing your Relationships
- Carving out TIME for Yourself and Your Loved Ones

Create the Life You Want to Live. Live by your Own Design.

Be Healthy, Be Happy, Be Well.

Additional Resources Follow to Maximize and Simplify your Path to Wellness Transformation.

Grocery Store List

When Planning Meals: Combine Protein, Fats and Complex Carbohydrates

Protein Options:

Tips: Choose lean meats. Choose organic, grass fed, cage free as much as possible. Focus on meatless options. Buy from local farms when possible. Eat small amounts of protein often.

Traditional Choices: Beef, chicken, turkey, veal, eggs, tuna, salmon, shrimp, cod, flounder, trout, halibut, lobster, scallops, crab, tofu or tempeh.

Beans: Black, soybean, kidney, green, chickpeas, hummus, green.

Nuts: All nuts and seeds and nut butters.

Dairy or Alternatives: Greek yogurt, Almond Milk, Rice Milk, Soy Milk, Cashew Milk, Hemp Milk, Coconut Milk, hard cheeses like parmesan and cheddar, feta, blue cheese, low fat cottage cheese.

Organic soy options: Kefir, kimchee, Greek Yogurt, natto, kombucha, miso, sauerkraut, fermented soy sauce, refrigerated pickles.

Healthy Fats:

Tip: Eat a small amount of healthy fat every time you eat.

Nuts: Almonds, brazil, walnuts, pecans, macadamia nuts, nut butters (peanut, almond, cashew, macadamia or walnut butter).

Seeds: Hemp, chia, flax, pumpkin, sesame, sunflower.

Oils: Coconut, olive, walnut, sesame, grapeseed, canola.

Other: Olives, avocado, butter, tahini, dark chocolate.

Complex Carbohydrates:

Tips: Make half your plate vegetables. Eat a variety of color every day and eat some raw and some cooked each day. Your goal is to include 5 different vegetables and 3 fruits every day. Breakfast should be 3 different fruits and a protein.

Focus on Greens: Kale, spinach, broccoli, Brussels sprouts, cabbage, arugula, asparagus, parsley, zucchini, Swiss chard, lettuces, cucumber, celery, artichoke, swiss chard, dandelion greens, collard greens, turnip greens, beet greens, bean sprouts, eggplant, chives, snow peas.

Other Vegetables: Sweet potato, squash, peppers, artichoke, carrots, garlic, zucchini, turnip, parsnips, rutabagas, cauliflower, mushrooms, onion, tomato, beets, eggplant, radishes, scallions.

Fruits: Strawberries, acai, pineapple, grapefruit, papaya, blackberry, raspberries, blueberries, lemon, lime, cherries, oranges, apples, banana, Goji berry, kiwi, grapes, prunes, pomegranate, watermelon, figs, dates, apricot, peach, pear, plum, tangerine.

Grains:

Rolled Oats, buckwheat, quinoa, millet, amaranth, brown rice, whole wheat pasta, whole wheat bread, barley, couscous.

Drinks:

Filtered water, green tea, lemon and ginger tea, all herbal teas and coffee.   *try not to drink calories

Spices/Seasonings:

Sea salt, black pepper, curry, thyme, rosemary, chili powder, cumin, sage, oregano, onion powder, cinnamon, paprika, parsley, basil, tomato sauce, mustard, horseradish, organic ketchup.

Healthy Snack Foods List

Oatmeal with fruit

Jell-O (with or without fruit)

Protein Bar

Whole wheat bagel with fat free cream cheese

Raw vegetables with yogurt based dip

Celery and peanut butter

Fresh fruit (apple, banana, grapes, grapefruit, oranges, melons, berries, kiwi, etc.)

Low fat yogurt with low fat granola

Pita bread with veggies and yogurt based dip

Low fat string cheese and apple

Whole grain cereal and almond milk

Soup (read labels…no soups with high sodium or processed meats in them)

Lean turkey, reduced fat cheese and whole wheat crackers

Turkey, sauerkraut and fruit

Soy chocolate oatmeal shake

Fruit smoothie

Green smoothie

Chocolate almond milk and peanut butter smoothie

Whole wheat pita pizza with low fat cheese and veggies

Brown rice, chilled with cinnamon and stevia

Whole grain cereal without milk

Pretzels (low salt) or rice cakes

Veggie Sandwich on whole wheat bread

Pita with hummus

Salads

Boiled egg and fruit

Grilled chicken breast

Avocado and turkey wrap

Trail Mix (nuts, seeds, chocolate chips and popcorn)

Dark Chocolate (grated and drizzled over fruit and whipped cream)

Oysters, sardines or tuna on a bed of lettuce

Salted edamame with olive oil and seasonings of your choice

Organic cheese and olives

Coconut milk and nut butter

Chickpeas with olive oil, lemon, salt, pepper

Dark chocolate covered almonds

Sprouted Grain bread with almond butter and spreadable fruit

Vegetable chips (slice thin, drizzle with olive oil, sea salt, pepper, parmesan)

Carrots, peppers, and hummus

Coconut milk ice cream with dark chocolate pieces

Overnight oats

Popcorn sprinkled with cinnamon, sea salt or 100% cocoa

Whole wheat pizza crust with asparagus, chicken and goat cheese or feta

Sample 3 Day Food Plan

DAY 1

BREAKFAST:

Water, and juice (acai, pomegranate, cherry or any super fruit blend)   (4-6 ounces of 100% juice)

Mixed fruit: A variety of whatever you like (fresh or frozen) ¾ to 1 cup total

Oranges, grapefruit, strawberries, blueberries, grapes, pineapple, cranberries

SNACK:

Water, tea or coffee

Oatmeal with raisins and brown sugar, cinnamon and organic 2% milk or milk alternative

1 slice of whole wheat toast with organic butter

LUNCH:

Water, tea or coffee

2 scrambled eggs loaded with veggies (onion, green/red/yellow peppers, tomato)

1 slice of whole grain toast with organic butter

SNACK:

Water, tea or coffee

Whole wheat pita with hummus. Add olive oil and parsley to the hummus

Carrots with a yogurt based dip

DINNER:

Water, decaf tea or coffee

Begin dinner with some raw broccoli and cauliflower

Grilled Steak

Green beans

SNACK:

Water or a nighttime blend of tea (no caffeine)

Coconut milk vanilla ice cream drizzled with dark chocolate

DAY 2

BREAKFAST:

Hot lemon water, green tea or coffee

Fruit Smoothie: blend together (a few ice cubes, 1 cup frozen cherries, 1/2 banana, 1 cup almond milk, ½ c. fat free plain or vanilla yogurt, 5 tsp. sliced almonds, 1 tablespoon pea protein powder)

SNACK:

Water, tea or coffee

High fiber cereal or oatmeal with blueberries and strawberries

LUNCH:

Water, tea or coffee

Whole wheat pita with fat free refried beans, low fat cheese, lettuce, tomato, tri-colored peppers and light sour cream.

SNACK:

Water, tea or coffee

Salad of mixed greens (add carrots, onion, celery, olives, feta, and pomegranate dressing)

DINNER:

Water, decaf tea or coffee

Grilled or Baked Chicken breast

Asparagus and natural applesauce with cinnamon

Sweet potatoes

SNACK:

Water or a nighttime blend of tea without caffeine

Whole wheat crackers with low fat cheese slices or hummus

Day 3

BREAKFAST:

Hot lemon water and cranberry juice (4-6 ounces)

Mixed fruit and organic granola (kiwi, peaches, raspberries, orange, grapefruit)

SNACK:

Water, tea or coffee

Celery, apple and peanut butter

5 pieces Dove Dark Chocolate with almonds

LUNCH:

Water, tea or coffee

Whole wheat pita or bread: turkey, sauerkraut, lettuce, tomato, low fat cheese, onion and horseradish or light mayo.

SNACK:

Water, tea or coffee

Mix of nuts and seeds ¼ cup total (cashews, walnuts, pecans, pistachio, sunflower seeds or pumpkins seeds) Add popcorn for more volume if you want

2 oz. of cheese (Swiss, mozzarella, cheddar, parmesan)

DINNER:

Water, decaf tea or coffee

Salad of mixed greens (add red cabbage, arugula, spinach, feta)

Salmon

Quinoa and stir fry mixture of vegetables

SNACK:

Water with splash of lime juice

Baked chips and salsa

Goal Setting Suggestions

1. My current fitness goal is:
   _____
   _____

2. My nutrition goal is:
   _____
   _____

3. My weight loss goal is: _____

   Hint: A realistic weight loss goal –divide your body weight by 100…that is the appropriate number of pounds to safely lose per week.

4. A personal short term goal –(in a month or less)
   _____
   _____

5. A personal long term goal-(in the next 5 years)
   _____
   _____

6. A professional short term goal- (in a month or less)
   _____
   _____

7. A professional long term goal-(in the next 5 years)
   _____
   _____

Tips for Effective Goal Setting:

- Write the goal down.
- Make is specific so that it can be measured.
- Include small action steps and a deadline.
- Share your goal with a friend. They can help with motivation and accountability.
- Be determined and committed to the goal. Do something daily toward goal achievement.
- Allow yourself the FEELING of what it will be like to reach that goal.
- Visualize it. Make a vison board or vison book of your goals.
- Feel it. Be enthusiastic and excited. Set a reward for achievement of the goal.

My Wishes for You

I Hope That You Will:

Treat yourself well.

Live every day as a gift.

Appreciate what you have.

Eliminate and manage stress.

Get enough sleep and relaxation.

Love with your whole heart and soul.

Create the life you long for and deserve.

Nourish your body with real, whole food.

Forgive yourself and others for everything.

Focus on your loved ones and be good to them.

Do what the average person doesn't want to do.

Make the decision to really live your life joyfully.

Seek joy, bliss, and laughter in your life every day.

Be there for the milestones in your children's lives.

Find a spiritual practice. Believe in a higher power.

Create your environment to be pleasing and calming.

End each day with meditation or journaling activities.

Set dreams and goals and fulfill them. Make memories.

Give of your time to others. Share your talents and gifts.

Exercise. Make movement part of your everyday routine.

Refuse to make decisions when you are upset or emotional.

Treat yourself at least as good as you would your best friend.

Remember that your happiness and fulfillment is in your hands.

Know when too much of a good thing is no longer a good thing.

Choose your words and actions wisely. Think before you speak.

Always do your best at everything you do. Always tell the truth.

Focus on yourself and be the designer and creator of a life you love.

Learn to ask for what you want and need. Develop a support system.

Begin each day by making positive affirmations. Use positive self-talk.

Do something every day that makes you feel good. Don't forget to play.

Use your energy wisely. Learn to say no. Delegate tasks when possible.

Splurge on these things: mattress, pillow, quality nutritious food and drinks.

Slow down and really look around you and enjoy each day as the gift that it is.

Live the life that you want to be remembered for. Most importantly, pay it forward.

God Bless You on your journey to focus on yourself and create a joyful existence.
It truly is up to you to live by your own design.
Best wishes for your health and happiness.

-Linda

INDEX

Acupuncture: 143
Acidic Foods: 98
Affirmations: 25
Air Quality: 138
Alternative Healing: 140
Alkaline Diet: 98
Anti-Aging: 112
Antioxidants: 78
Artificial Sweeteners: 72
Aromatherapy: 141
Ayurveda: 144
Beans: 58
Blood Type: 155
Breakfast: 90, 92
Brain Health: 112
Breathing: 106
Calming: 106
Calorie Burning: 64, 84
Carbohydrates: 57
Cardio: 44
Causes of Disease: 95
Chiropractic: 140
Clean Eating: 38
Commitment: 21
Condiments: 101
Contentment: 159
Cravings: 38
Cruciferous Foods: 80
Dairy Alternatives: 37
Dehydration: 47
Determination: 22
Detoxification: 149
Diagnostic Tests: 50
Digestion: 61
Dining Out: 132
Disease Prevention: 95
Distance: 46
Drinks: 37, 175
Environment: 137
Essential Oils: 99, 142
Fats: 54

Fat Burning: 81
Fermented Foods: 66
Fiber: 58
Fit for Life: 55
Fitness: 42, 59, 81, 106, 134, 155
Fitness Assessments: 134
Fitness Goals: 44
Food Plan: 178
Food and Mood: 65
Foods and Water Content: 48
Forgiveness: 103
Functional Fitnes: 156
Gluten: 62, 75
Gluten Sensitivity: 62
Goal Refinement: 163
Goal Setting: 29, 163, 181
Grains: 75
Gratitude: 60
Greens: 49
Grocery Shopping: 89, 174
Grocery Store List: 174
Guided Imagery: 109
Guidelines for Fitness: 42
Happiness: 120
Health Boosts: 91
Health Commandments: 23
Health Tips: 72
Healthy Fats: 54
Healthy Snack Foods: 176
Herbal Medicine: 144
Homeopathy: 143
Holistic: 173
Home Cooking: 88
Hunger Scale: 64
Hydration: 47
Immune Boosting: 78
Individualized Plan: 154
Inflammation: 96, 97
Inspiration: 9
Interval Training: 82
Journaling: 84

Joy: 159
Kitchen Basics: 36
Kitchen Clean Up: 35
Label Reading: 35
Legumes: 71
Logging Methods: 46, 70, 73
Life Purpose: 160
Life Review: 163
Life Satisfaction Survey: 28
Living Food: 36, 80
Malnourished: 96
Massage: 141
Meal Planning: 89, 178-180
Meal Preparation: 89
Meditation: 107
Motivation: 21
MUFA: 55
My Wishes for You: 183
Nature: 103
Nitrates: 36, 54
Numbers to Know: 135
Oils: 37
Omega 3: 97
Omega 6: 97
Organic: 89, 114, 149
Overnight Oats: 91
Overweight: 96
Passion: 159
Personal Information: 135
Personal Mission Statement: 161
Physical Environment: 137
Phytonutrients: 78
Planning: 39
Plants: 138
Polarity: 145
Portion Control: 130
Pranic Healing: 145
Prebiotic: 63
Preparation: 39
Priorities: 157
Probiotic: 62
Progressive Relaxation: 108
Promises: 22
Protein: 53

Protein Bars: 54
Protein Powder: 53
Purpose: 159
Raw Food Diet: 80
Real Age: 112
Real Food: 36, 80
Recipes: 76, 77, 90, 91
Reiki: 145
Regret: 105
Relationships: 150-153
Resentment: 105
Responsibilities: 158
Rewards: 29
Roles: 158
Routine: 39, 41
Seasonings: 175
Serving Sizes: 130
Simplicity: 39, 41
Skin Care: 112
Sleep: 127
Soy: 56
Spices: 63, 100, 101, 175
Spirituality: 102
Smoothies: 90
Strength: 59
Stress: 114
Success Tips: 22
Super Foods: 78
Super Greens: 50, 97
Supplements: 66
Sweeteners: 37
Target Heart Rate: 46
Teas: 100
Teeth Whitening: 114
Ten Health Commandments: 23
Time: 40, 157
Time Management: 157
Time Saving Tips: 40
Tips for Success: 22
Toxic Foods: 36
Toxins: 138
Trans Fats: 56
Ultimate Health: 69
Ultimate Health Food Diary: 70

Ultimate Health Food Tips: 72
Vegetarian: 54
Water: 47
Weight Loss: 64
Weight Training: 59
Wish List: 168
Yoga: 107

Made in the USA
Lexington, KY
07 May 2017